Davenport

The Osteoporotic Syndrome

The Osteoporotic Syndrome
Detection, Prevention, and Treatment

Edited by

Louis V. Avioli, M.D.

Schoenberg Professor of Medicine
Director, Division of Bone and Mineral Metabolism
Washington University School of Medicine
The Jewish Hospital of St. Louis
St. Louis, Missouri

Grune & Stratton
A Subsidiary of Harcourt Brace Jovanovich, Publishers
New York   London
Paris   San Diego   San Francisco   São Paulo
Sydney   Tokyo   Toronto

Library of Congress Cataloging in Publication Data

Main entry under title:

The Osteoporotic syndrome.

Bibliography: p.
Includes index.
1. Osteoporosis.   2. Osteoporosis—Age factors.
3. Women—Diseases.   I. Avioli, Louis V.   [DNLM:
1. Osteoporosis.   WE 250 0867]
RC931.O73079   1983   616.7'1   83-8854
ISBN 0-8089-1548-7

© 1983 by Grune and Stratton, Inc.
All rights reserved. No part of this publication
may be reproduced or transmitted in any form or
by any means, electronic or mechanical, including
photocopy, recording, or any information storage
and retrieval system, without permission in
writing from the publisher.

Grune & Stratton, Inc.
111 Fifth Avenue
New York, New York 10003

Distributed in the United Kingdom by
Academic Press Inc. (London) Ltd.
24/28 Oval Road, London NW 1

Library of Congress Catalog Number 83-8854
International Standard Book Number 0-8089-1548-7
Printed in the United States of America

Contents

Preface   *vii*

Contributors   *ix*

1 The Menopausal Patient
B. E. C. Nordin   *1*

2 Osteoporosis with Particular Reference to the Menopause
B. E. C. Nordin   *13*

3 Epidemiology of Age-related Fractures
L. Joseph Melton, III, and B. Lawrence Riggs   *45*

4 Noninvasive Methods for Quantitating Appendicular Bone Mass
C. Conrad Johnston, Jr.   *73*

5 Noninvasive Methods for Quantitating Trabecular Bone
Richard B. Mazess   *85*

6 Osteoporosis and the Bone Biopsy
Steven L. Teitelbaum   *115*

7 Prevention of Age-related Osteoporosis in Women
Robert P. Heaney   *123*

8 The Management of the Geriatric Osteoporotic Woman
Louis V. Avioli   *145*

Index   *155*

Preface

Our aging population is steadily increasing in number, and the majority are women predisposed to an osteoporotic fracture syndrome. Thus, physicians should become familiar with techniques currently available to detect those patients at risk and the manner by which the relentless bone loss can be effectively abated.

There is a disproportionate increased incidence of skeletal fracture in the aging female. Clinicians must be concerned with the morbidity and cost accountability of the bone-fracture syndrome, and confront the simple questions that necessarily result from a plethora of well-documented facts: Why is it that all postmenopausal women do not develop a dowager's hump, an anatomic change that reflects the rapid loss of vertebral bone mass? What factors predispose some postmenopausal women to a greater incidence of vertebral, forearm, and femoral neck fractures? Is the underlying pathogenesis identical and the bone loss uniform for all postmenopausal women who are destined for more rapid bone loss and early fractures? What changes in hormonal and mineral metabolism necessarily result from senescence in females, and how are they related to the loss of bone? Are the effects of aging on bone similar in men and women and, if so, why are women more predisposed to fractures? To what extent can we honestly believe that our present techniques are sufficiently sensitive to allow firm convictions with respect to those hormonal, metabolic, and skeletal alterations that accompany the aging process? Should we not examine and reevaluate available data regarding dietary intake, recommended dietary allowances, as well as the need and potential hazards of hormonal replacement in the peri- and postmenopausal female?

It is now accepted that bone mass reaches its apogee in all individuals sometime within the third and fourth decades of life. Although we recognize that bone loss (primarily vertebral) continues thereafter, it has not been conclusively established that all humans lose bone with age. In fact, there are data that demonstrate that bone loss does not occur with age in some individuals. Yet, given the fact that bone loss occurs with age in the majority of individuals, what mechanisms can be presently invoked to account for this delay? Advocates of acquired alterations in ovarian hormonal secretion and/or metabolism often cite a variety of factors: (1) data regarding the more rapid loss of bone in females than males, (2) accelerated loss of bone in females in their postmenopausal years, (3) increased fracture incidence in females with congenital disturbances in ovarian function, and (4) salutary skeletal responses of postmenopausal females to estrogen "replacement" therapy.

Recent observations illustrating the progressive loss of vertebral bone in women beginning in the third and fourth decades of life, when ovarian function and blood estrogens are presumably normal, warrant specific attention. Surely, the progressive loss of bone that occurs in the young, ovulating female cannot be attributed to alterations in estrogen release and metabolism! What factors condition this loss of skeletal mass, and are they related to a deficiency in dietary calcium? Moreover, is it possible to extrapolate from data accumulated in peri- and postmenopausal females who present with abnormally low calcium intakes and/or defective calcium utilization and who respond to dietary calcium supplementation with a retardation in the rate of bone loss? These and other questions are addressed in this monograph. The combined analyses of the "osteoporotic problem" by the present group of clinicians and scientists should offer the practicing physician a definitive and rational approach to the diagnosis and therapy of osteoporosis in the aging female. When the osteoporotic syndrome is examined as a progressive, subtle, and potentially remedial process that characterizes the third, fourth, and fifth decades of life in the female, the ravages and morbidity of the syndrome observed in the postmenopausal population are seen to be preventable to a considerable degree.

Contributors

Louis V. Avioli, M.D.
Schoenberg Professor of Medicine
Director, Division of Bone and Mineral Metabolism
Washington University School of Medicine
The Jewish Hospital of St. Louis
St. Louis, Missouri

Robert P. Heaney, M.D.
Professor of Medicine
Vice President for Health Sciences
Creighton University
Omaha, Nebraska

C. Conrad Johnston, Jr., M.D.
Professor of Medicine
Director, Division of Endocrinology and Metabolism
Indiana University
Indianapolis, Indiana

Richard B. Mazess, Ph.D.
Associate Professor of Medical Physics
University of Wisconsin
Madison, Wisconsin

L. Joseph Melton, III, M.D.
Associate Professor of Epidemiology
Mayo Medical School
Rochester, Minnesota

B.E.C. Nordin, M.D., F.R.C.P., D.Sc.
Clinical Professor, Endocrine Unit
Royal Adelaide Hospital
North Terrace, Adelaide
South Australia

B. Lawrence Riggs, M.D.
Professor of Medicine
Chairman, Division of Endocrinology and Metabolism
Mayo Medical School
Rochester, Minnesota

Steven L. Teitelbaum, M.D.
Professor of Pathology
Washington University School of Medicine
The Jewish Hospital of St. Louis
St. Louis, Missouri

1

The Menopausal Patient

B. E. C. Nordin

DEFINITION OF THE MENOPAUSE

Throughout reproductive life, a normal woman sheds the lining of her uterus about once every 28 days. This endometrial shedding is the result of a cyclical hormonal pattern that involves estrogen-induced proliferation of the endometrium during the first half of the month (the proliferative phase), which leads up to ovulation at midcycle. In the second half of the month, the combined effects of estrogen and progesterone (secreted by the corpus luteum that develops after ovulation) transform the endometrium to a secretory state. At the end of the month (unless conception has occurred) the estrogen and progesterone levels fall and the endometrium is shed.

As the number of available primordial follicules declines, generally in the fifth decade of life, anovular and irregular cycles begin to occur until menstruation finally ceases at an average of 48 to 49 years. The menopause is dated from this last menstrual cycle, but owing to the irregularity of cycles around this time it can only be clearly defined in retrospect—sometimes a woman has a solitary menstrual bleed six months, one year, or even longer after what she thought was her last menstruation—and it is, therefore, generally agreed that at least one year without bleeding must elapse before the menopause can be said to have occurred. It is then dated from the last menstrual period.

Although the mean age at menopause is about 48 to 49 years in the Western world, the age range is wide. By definition, 50 percent of women reach the menopause before that age and 50 percent after it, but 2 to 3 percent become menopausal before the age of 40, and there are a

1

few women whose menstruation ceases before the age of 30. At the other end of the scale, the menopause seldom extends beyond 56 years. The situation is further complicated by the increasing proportion of women who undergo a surgical menopause (now something like 30 percent or even more), in some of whom the ovaries are removed while in others they are conserved. Simple hysterectomy with conservation of the ovaries (or sometimes one ovary) gives rise to an apparent menopause in that menstruation ceases but does not cause the hormonal changes, nor generally gives rise to the symptoms, associated with the true menopause unless, of course, the ovaries or their blood supply are damaged in the operation. Ovariectomy, on the other hand (with or without hysterectomy), produces the real equivalent of a menopause, though very much more abruptly than occurs in the normal situation and often with more severe symptomatology. Thus, although the menopause is defined for clinical purposes by the occurrence of the last menstrual period, it is probably more rational to define it in hormonal terms. When this is done as described below, it is found that some women who are still menstruating (albeit irregularly) are really postmenopausal in the hormonal sense, whereas others who have not menstruated for a year, or occasionally even longer, are still hormonally premenopausal.

HORMONAL EVENTS

The menopause is associated with an abrupt decline in the main plasma estrogens, estradiol and estrone, and a reciprocal rise in the plasma levels of the gonadotrophins—follicle stimulating hormone (FSH) and luteinising hormone (LH).

The plasma estradiol (E_2) levels in regularly menstruating premenopausal women and in unequivocally postmenopausal ovariectomized women are shown in Figure 1-1. There is no overlap between them. All the premenopausal women have plasma levels over 100 pmol/l, and all the ovariectomized women have values below 60 pmol/l. It is thus generally possible to establish whether a woman is hormonally pre- or postmenopausal by a single measurement of plasma estradiol despite the wide variation in its value during the menstrual cycle. Occasionally, however, in perimenopausal women with irregular menses, intermediate values between 60 and 100 pmol/l do occur, and the cor-

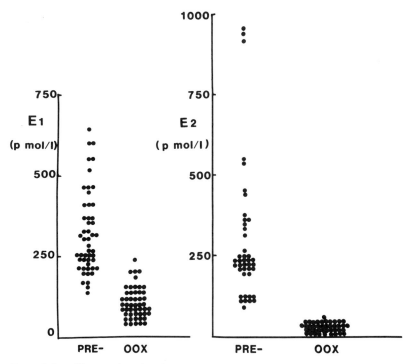

Fig. 1-1. Plasma levels of estrone (left) and estradiol (right) in pre-menopausal women with regular menstruation, and in oophorec-tomized women.

rect classification in these cases must then depend upon the simultane-ous measurement of FSH (see below).

Plasma estrone (E_1) levels in pre- and postmenopausal women are also shown in Figure 1-1. The premenopausal mean is clearly much higher than the postmenopausal mean, but there is considerable overlap between the two groups in the region of 100 to 200 pmol/l. Moreover, the proportionate fall in plasma estrone is not nearly as great as that in plasma estradiol, and whereas the premenopausal plasma estrone is lower than the estradiol level, in postmenopausal women the plasma estrone is higher than the estradiol. The reason for this is that plasma estrone is not only secreted by the ovary but can be derived by periph-eral conversion from the weak androgen androstenedione, which is se-creted not only by the ovaries but also by the adrenals. The menopau-

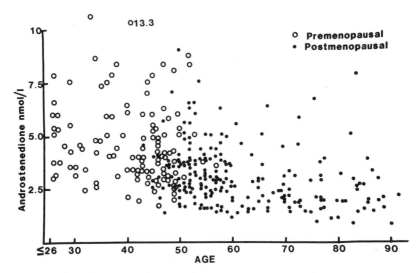

Fig. 1-2.   Plasma androstenedione levels in pre- and postmenopausal women.

sal fall in plasma estrone therefore only represents a fall in the ovarian contribution, which represents about 50 percent of the total, with the result that high postmenopausal values overlap with the low premenopausal values. Estrone is, therefore, the dominant estrogen in the postmenopausal woman in the quantitative sense. Because it is less potent than estradiol; however, the relative contributions of the two to the hormonal status of the postmenopausal woman has not been fully elucidated.

Because of the ovarian follicular secretion of androstenedione (which is also cyclical), at menopause there is also a fall in the plasma level of about 50 percent of this weak androgen (Fig. 1-2). Thus the residual plasma androstenedione in the postmenopausal woman represents adrenal secretion only. It is rather lower than in men because males can also derive androstenedione from peripheral conversion from testosterone.

There are striking reciprocal changes in the plasma gonadotrophin levels as shown in Figure 1-3. There is no overlap in plasma FSH levels between truly premenopausal and postmenopausal women; they are always below 20 units/1 in the premenopausal woman and above 30 units/1 in the postmenopausal woman. During the perimenopausal period, however, intermediate values may be observed and the true classi-

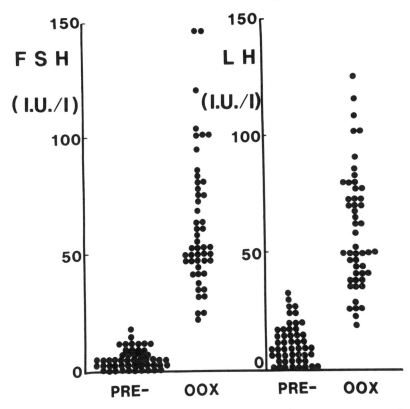

Fig. 1-3. Plasma levels of FSH (left) and LH (right) in premenopausal and oophorectomized women.

fication of the patient then requires a plasma estradiol measurement (see below). Plasma LH levels also rise, but there remains a significant overlap between pre- and postmenopausal values (Fig. 1-3).

The reciprocal relationship between plasma estradiol and FSH in unselected pre- and postmenopausal women when the data are combined is shown in Figure 1-4. The double lines on the vertical and horizontal axes embrace the equivocal ranges within which it may be necessary to perform both estimations to classify the patient correctly. It is clear that there are a few patients who combine a high FSH with a high plasma estradiol level; these cases defy classification. Patients who combine low FSH levels with low plasma estradiol are either suffering from pituitary insufficiency or are taking the contraceptive pill; no such cases are shown in Figure 1-4.

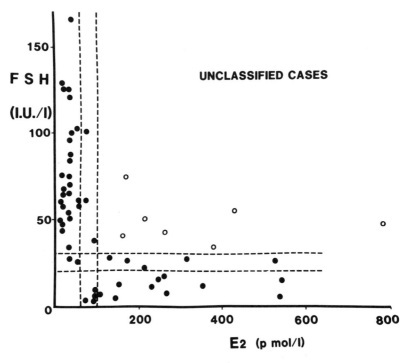

Fig. 1-4. Relationship between plasma estradiol and FSH levels in unselected women attending a menopause clinic. The interrupted lines embrace the equivocal zone of each variable. The seven patients with open circles represent cases who cannot be classified into the pre- or postmenopausal groups.

SYMPTOMATOLOGY

Varied symptoms are associated with and have been attributed to the menopause. The application of discriminant function analysis to the symptoms complained of by pre- and postmenopausal women shows that the most powerful discriminant between them is the hot flush, which is a sensation of heat affecting the upper part of the body that may occur spontaneously or be triggered by an emotional stimulus. The flush is frequently followed by a sweat, particularly at night. As the syndrome evolves, however, the flush becomes less and less marked and the sweats become more and more dominant. Most (though not all) women suffer from some degree of flushing at the menopause, varying from an occasional weekly flush to flushes many, many times a day and several sweating attacks during the night. The natural history of this complaint is extremely variable, however. In most women it is self-limiting and lasts one to five years, but in a minority it continues for much longer, and we have known patients still complaining of flushes in the eighth decade. The mechanism of the flushes is unknown, but they tend to be more prevalent in the patients with the highest plasma gonadotrophin levels.

The second most common symptom of the menopause is a decline in libido, usually associated with reduced vaginal secretion, which is occasionally severe enough to cause dyspareunia. This loss of sexual interest may seriously jeopardize what was previously a harmonious, marital relationship.

The third most important symptom is a loss of confidence that may express itself as anxiety and/or depression and sometimes compels a successful, professional woman to give up her occupation.

There are many other symptoms that seem to occur more commonly in perimenopausal women than at other times of life, but their causal connection with the menopause is uncertain. They include headaches, insomnia, arthralgias, and others too numerous to mention. These symptoms should be treated with some reserve unless associated with hot flushes.

TREATMENT

Indications

The most specific symptom of the menopause is the hot flush, and it is, therefore, not surprisingly the one that responds most satisfactorily to hormonal treatment. Whether it requires treatment will depend on its frequency and severity and its association with other menopausal complaints, which frequently subside when the hot flush is controlled. Hot flushes in isolation (a rather unusual situation) are not worth treating unless the patient finds them very disabling. They are, however, an extremely useful marker that tells the physician that the patient's other complaints are likely to be menopausal in origin and may improve on therapy.

When reduced sexuality occurs at or about the time of the menopause, it can be regarded as an indication for estrogen therapy, or at least for a prolonged trial of estrogen therapy, even when the hot flushes are absent or minimal. Vaginal dryness and/or dyspareunia are particularly strong indications for estrogen therapy at this time of life.

Loss of confidence (and all that this implies) is an indication for estrogen therapy if associated with flushes and/or vaginal dryness. When it occurs in the perimenopausal period, loss of confidence in isolation merits a trial on estrogen therapy for a short period only.

The other more nebulous symptoms of the menopause are unlikely to respond to estrogen therapy unless they are associated with one or more of the above three cardinal symptoms.

Dosage Regimens

The object of therapy should be to use the smallest dose of estrogen that will control the symptoms. One should therefore start with a low dose and increase it at monthly intervals if necessary. Starting doses are 0.3 mg of conjugated estrogens, 1 mg of estradiol valerate, 1.5 mg of estrone piperizime sulphate, or 10 μg of ethinyl estradiol. Despite the widespread concern about endometrial cancer, progestogen therapy is not mandatory provided that the estrogen is given in a small dose on a cyclical basis for three weeks out of four and the patient is kept under regular observation. However, in perimenopausal women, *i.e.* those who are still menstruating, albeit irregularly, a cyclical progestogen should be included in the regime—generally norethisterone 5 mg daily for the third week of the three-week cycle. A progestogen should also be added for any patient in whom bleeding is delayed or extends into the first week of the next cycle or occurs at any other inappropriate time. Frequently, the most appropriate regime for young perimenopausal women is a cyclical preparation (Menophase), which is a monthly pack of estrogen (methyl ethinyl estradiol) and progesterone (Levo Norgestrel) in graded doses. The three weeks out of four regime should be observed even in hysterectomized women, because although estrogen therapy has not been implicated in the genesis of breast cancer, one does not wish to incur any risk of overstimulation of the breast.

In cases where estrogens are contraindicated and the indications for hormone therapy are strong, norethisterone 5 mg daily should be used continuously. Although not quite as effective as estrogens in controlling menopausal symptoms, it is an excellent second best and has an excellent safety record. It should be noted, however, that in any woman with a proliferative endometrium (for instance, one who has previously taken estrogen therapy) norethisterone may induce bleeding. This bleeding episode will only occur once and does not recur once the endometrium has been shed. It is, therefore, a wise precaution to give norethisterone initially for a three-week period to any woman with an intact uterus and then allow a week for bleeding before continuous norethisterone therapy is commenced. If bleeding occurs during this first three-week period, the patient should be instructed to stop norethisterone and not resume it until the bleeding has stopped; it can be given continuously from that time onward.

Contraindications to Estrogen Therapy

Estrogens should not be administered to women who have had endometrial cancer or breast cancer, to women with proven ischemic heart disease, to those with bad varicose veins, or to any woman with a past history of thromboembolic disease or very severe varicose veins. In these patients, therapy can be substituted as described above.

Duration of Therapy

It is impossible to lay down any firm rules for the duration of estrogen therapy. As with all other treatment, it should be continued for as long as it appears to benefit the patient, though seldom beyond the age of 65. The menopausal syndrome is essentially self-limiting, and treatment is designed to cover the natural history of the disorder. Sometimes the patient herself will suggest that she would like to try going without hormones for a month or two. In some of these women the symptoms recur and the treatment has to be reinstituted; in others this is not the case. Sometimes it is the doctor who suggests that treatment has gone on for long enough and should be discontinued for a trial period. Sometimes it is necessary to stop it because angina or coronary heart disease, which was probably pre-existing, becomes manifest. Occasionally, treatment is discontinued because of nausea or breast tenderness when all that is required is a reduction in dosage. Treatment should, however, be discontinued, at least temporarily, if the patient is to undergo a surgical operation or is for any other reason confined to bed for any length of time.

Response to Treatment

Hot flushes and sweats are almost invariably controlled by estrogen therapy in about two weeks if the dose is adequate. Vaginal dryness and dyspareunia are generally corrected quite quickly, but impaired libido does not always respond to therapy or may take some months to recover. There is generally a striking improvement in self-confidence in those patients where this has been a major complaint. The other symptoms that are more loosely connected with the menopause, such as the arthralgias, respond in a rather unpredictable manner.

In addition to the control of symptoms, estrogen therapy does have beneficial effects on bone. The best documented of these is the control of bone resorption and consequent inhibition of bone loss (see Chapters 7 and 8). It should be emphasized, however, that long-term commitments with large doses of conjugated estrogens designed to achieve this purpose should be attempted with caution because of documented increased incidence of endometrial carcinoma in patients treated as such. Small-dose estrogen therapy with intermittent use of progestional agents is recommended in this regard. Moreover, appropriate clinical and cytologic analyses of the uterus should be obtained routinely whenever this form of treatment is initiated.

CONCLUSIONS

The menopause involves major hormonal changes that give rise to a variety of symptoms. Although there is very little correlation between the hormonal levels in postmenopausal women and the severity of their symptoms, the latter generally respond to hormone therapy. In most cases, however, this can hardly be regarded as "replacement therapy" analogous to replacement with other hormones such as thyroid hormone, since the menopausal syndrome is a self-limiting disorder. Unlike replacement therapy with other hormones, estrogen treatment for menopausal symptoms need not continue indefinitely. It could be said that the menopausal syndrome is a manifestation of relative rather than absolute estrogen deficiency.

Nonetheless, there is probably a syndrome of true estrogen deficiency that affects postmenopausal women with the lowest estrogen levels. It is from this population that the cases with the most severe tissue changes (osteoporosis, vaginal atrophy, and possibly ischemic heart disease) are recruited, and it may be that the time is approaching when the patients in this category (who do not necessarily have the most severe menopausal complaints) will be identified by plasma hormone assays before tissue damage has occurred and treated with long-term, low-dose estrogen-progesterone regimens. This state of affairs has not yet arrived, and in the meantime short-term estrogen therapy is generally used to control the self-limiting menopausal syndrome.

BIBLIOGRAPHY

Avioli LV: Aging bone and osteoporosis, in Korenman SC (ed): *Endocrine Aspects of Aging.* New York, Elsevier Biomedical, Exford, 1982, pp 199–230

Casper R, Yen S, Wilkes, M: Menopausal flushes: A neuroendocrine link with pulsatile luteinizing hormone secretion. Science 205:823–825, 1979

DeFazio J, Meldrum DK, Laufer L, Vale W, Rivier J, Lu JKH, Judd HL: Induction of hot flushes in premenopausal women treated with a long-acting GNRH agonist. J Clin Endocrinol Metab 56:445–448, 1982

Erlik Y, Meldrum DR, Judd HL: Estrogen levels in postmenopausal women with hot flashes. J Am Col Obstet Gynecol 59:403–407, 1982

Hammond C, Maxson W: Current status of estrogen therapy for the menopause. Modern Trends 37:5–25, 1982

Hutton JD, Murray M, Jacobs H, James V: Relation between plasma estrone and estradiol and climacteric symptoms. Lancet 1:678–681, 1978

Judd H, Cleary R, Creasman W, Figge D, Kase N, Rosenwaks Z, Tagatz G: Estrogen replacement therapy. Obstet Gynecol 58:267–275, 1981

Judd H, Meldrum DR, Deftos LJ, Henderson BE: Estrogen replacement therapy: indications and complications. Ann Intern Med 98:195–205, 1982

Notelovitz M: When and how to use estrogen therapy in women over 60. Geriatrics 113–124, 1980

2

Osteoporosis with Particular Reference to the Menopause

B. E. C. Nordin

DEFINITION AND DIAGNOSIS

Osteoporosis denotes a reduced amount of bone. The chemical composition of the bone is unchanged; there is simply less of it. In trabecular bone, the trabeculae are abnormally thin and sparse; in cortical bone, the cortical width is reduced and the haversian canals are enlarged. Osteoporosis must be distinguished from osteomalacia, in which the amount of bone may be normal but its mineral content is reduced. Osteoporosis is due to increased breakdown or reduced formation of *whole bone;* osteomalacia is due to delayed mineralization of new bone. Densitometric procedures that rely on the radio density of calcium phosphate cannot, strictly speaking, distinguish between osteoporosis (reduced mineral and matrix) and osteomalacia (reduced mineral only), but because the latter condition is relatively rare, confusion seldom arises (see Chapters 4 and 5).

In quantitative terms, a bone is osteoporotic when the volume of tissue per unit volume of anatomic bone (volume/volume ratio) falls below the lower normal limit in young adults. If the value is within the normal range for the age and sex of the subject, simple osteoporosis is present; if it is below the range for age and sex, accelerated osteoporosis is present. Cortical and trabecular bone do not behave in exactly the same way, however, so it is necessary to define cortical and trabecular bone status independently in any given case. Cortical bone status is easily defined; and cortical osteoporosis is easily diagnosed on a plain

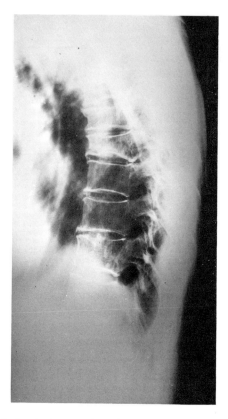

Fig. 2-1. Lateral thoracic breathing spine in a case of early osteoporosis. Note one wedged vertebra.

hand radiograph (as described below), but trabecular bone status is harder to define and ideally requires a bone biopsy. In clinical practice, osteoporosis is diagnosed from radiographs, and for this purpose a standard set of films should be taken. They should comprise a lateral breathing thoracic spine (to eliminate lung markings), a lateral lumbar spine, a full pelvis with proximal femora, and contact films of both hands. The spine films are examined for the following features:

1. *Radiolucency of the vertebrae.* Although this is subject to exposure factors, it is possible with experience and with good films to form some estimate of the apparent "density" of the vertebrae by masking the cortical outline of a vertebra and deciding whether the vertebral body would have been distinguishable from the soft tissue background if the cortex had not been present. If not, there has already been substantial loss of trabecular bone. If the iliac crest

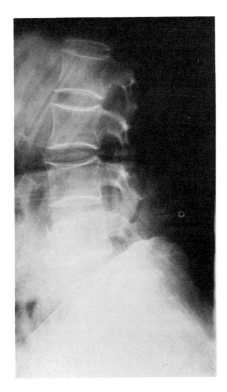

Fig. 2-2. Lateral lumbar spine in a case of early osteoporosis. Note translucency of the vertebrae and mild biconcavity.

can be clearly defined through the fourth or fifth lumbar vertebra, this is further evidence of reduced "density" (Figs. 2-1 and 2-2).

2. *Vertical trabeculation.* In the development of vertebral osteoporosis, the horizontal trabeculae are lost preferentially before the vertical trabeculae and the consequent accentuation of the latter can be taken as a sign of early osteoporosis.

3. *Biconcavity.* Vertebral biconcavity is an important indicator of osteoporosis, particularly in younger cases in whom the turgid intervertebral discs expand into the vertebral bodies (Figs. 2-1 and 2-2). It is less frequently seen in older cases when the discs have degenerated.

4. *Wedging.* If the anterior height of the vertebra is less than the posterior height, wedging is present. One wedged vertebra may simply denote previous trauma, but several wedged vertebrae indicate some degree of osteoporosis. Wedging occurs predominantly in the thoracic spine (Fig. 2-1).

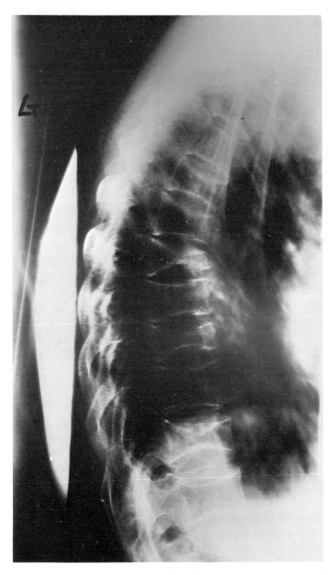

Fig. 2-3. Lateral thoracic breathing spine in a case of severe osteoporosis. Note multiple wedging and compression.

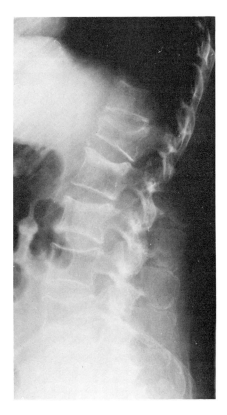

Fig. 2-4. Lateral lumbar spine in a case of severe osteoporosis. Note irregular deformation of the vertebrae.

5. *Compression.* A single compressed vertebra may simply be the result of trauma to a mildly osteoporotic spine, but the presence of two or more compressed vertebrae almost invariably indicates the presence of accelerated osteoporosis, i.e., a degree of osteoporosis excessive for the age of the patient (Figs. 2-3 and 2-4). (Compression is present when both the posterior and anterior heights of the vertebra are reduced.)

The radiological appearances of spinal osteoporosis may be completely mimicked by myelomatosis, and this diagnosis must always be excluded before osteoporosis as such is diagnosed. Secondary metastases from breast or other primaries may also cause compressed vertebrae but, when this is the cause, the rest of the spine generally looks normal—unless of course metastases and osteoporosis are present at the same time.

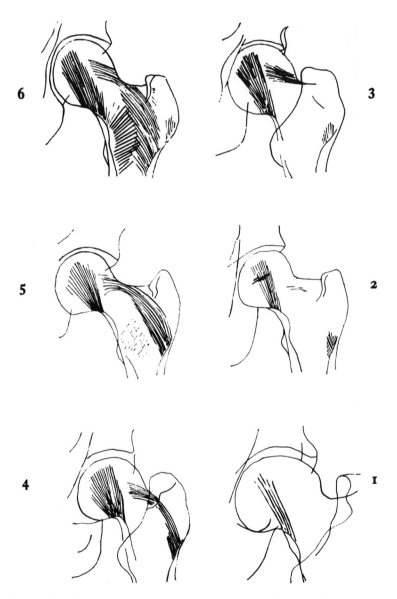

Fig. 2-5. Diagrammatic representation of the Singh index. Note the progressive loss of trabeculae at lower index values.

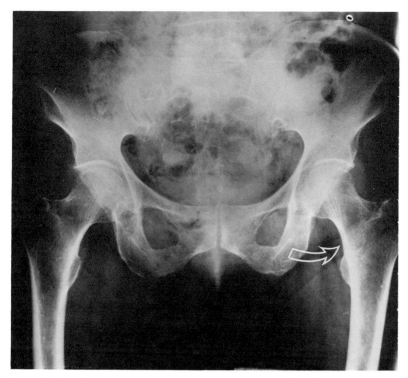

Fig. 2-6. Radiograph of the pelvis in a case of mild osteoporosis showing thick calcar femorale (indicated by arrow) and Singh index of about 4.

The pelvic film should be examined from the following points of view:

1. *The Singh index.* The Singh index represents only an approximation of the trabecular bone status in the proximal femur, which is graded on a six-point scale (Fig. 2-5). Values of 3 or less carry a greatly increased risk of femoral neck fracture. The Singh index may be reduced in groups of patients with vertebral compression and in cases of distal forearm fracture and femoral neck fracture, but it is often normal in individual cases (Figs. 2-6–2-10).

2. *Calcar femorale.* The thickness of the calcar femorale (the condensation of cortical bone immediately above the lesser trochanter) is significantly related to femoral neck fracture risk, and is generally

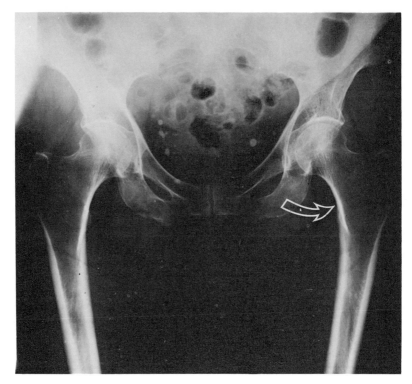

Fig. 2-7.   Pelvic radiograph in a case of severe osteoporosis. Note the thin calcar femorale (indicated by arrow) and a Singh index of about 2.

over 5 mm in normal subjects, and below this value in femoral neck fracture cases (Fig. 2-11).

Hands

Medullary width (MW) and total width (TW) are measured at the midpoint of the second metacarpal of the right hand (preferably with needle calipers). The difference between them represents cortical width (CW). The best measure of cortical bone status is the ratio of cortical area (CA) to total area (TA), which is calculated from the following simple formula:

$$CA/TA = \frac{TW^2 - MW^2}{TW^2}$$

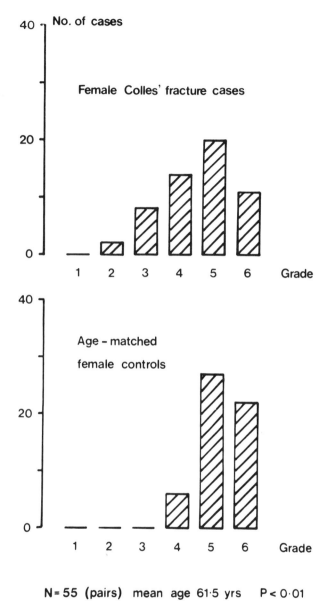

N = 55 (pairs) mean age 61·5 yrs   P < 0·01

Fig. 2-8. Frequency distribution histograms of the Singh index in 55 age-matched wrist fracture cases (top) and controls (below). Note the excess of low Singh index values in the fracture cases.

21

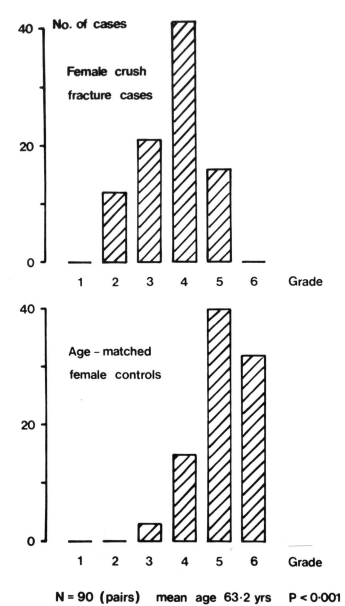

N = 90 (pairs)   mean age 63·2 yrs   P < 0·001

Fig. 2-9. Frequency distribution histograms of Singh index in female crush fracture cases (top) and age-matched controls (below). Note the excess of low values in the fracture cases.

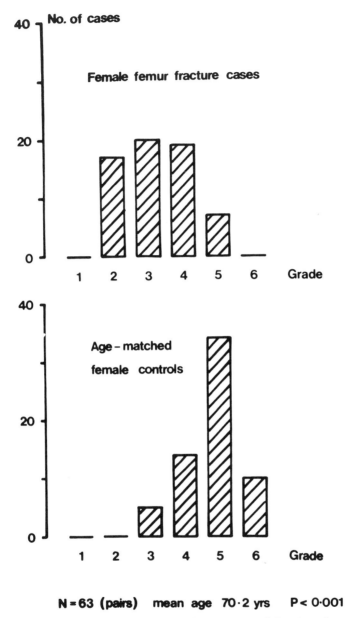

N = 63 (pairs)   mean age 70·2 yrs   P < 0·001

Fig. 2-10. Frequency distribution histograms of Singh index in female femur fracture cases (top) and age-matched controls (below). Note the great excess of low values in the fracture cases.

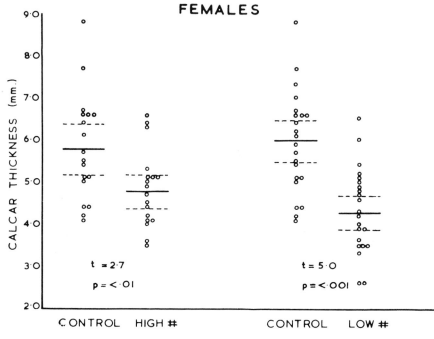

Fig. 2-11. Calcar femorale thickness in high femoral neck fracture cases and age-matched controls (left) and per-trochanteric fractures and age-matched controls (right). Note the reduced calcar thickness in both types of fracture.

The mean value of CA/TA in young adults is about 0.85 with a lower limit of 0.72, and it falls with age, more rapidly in women than men (Fig. 2-12) and values below 0.72 represent cortical osteoporosis. If the value is below the lower normal limit for age and sex, the patient has accelerated cortical osteoporosis (Fig. 2-13). Fracture cases as *groups* have reduced CA/TA values, although many *individuals* fall within the normal range for their age (Fig. 2-14).

The definition of cortical bone status is more precise than that of trabecular bone status, although the latter is more important in clinical practice (at least in the middle-aged population) because the risk of fracture of the vertebrae, wrist, and femoral neck is greatly increased by trabecular bone loss, which is itself much more rapid in middle age

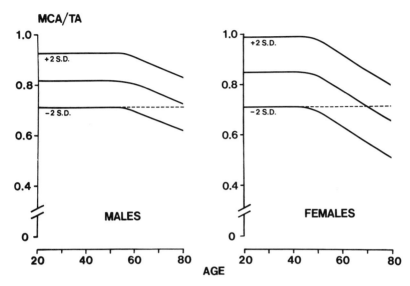

Fig. 2-12. Metacarpal cortical-area/total-area ratios as a function of age in normal males and females. Note that with advancing age an increasing proportion of the population fall below the young normal lower limit.

than the corresponding loss of cortical bone (see below). In major centers, trabecular bone densitometry by computerized axial tomography or by photon absorptiometry is becoming increasingly available. The limitations and diagnostic efficiency of these noninvasive techniques are detailed in Chapters 4 and 5. These techniques make it possible to diagnose trabecular osteoporosis with confidence before fracture has occurred. Without them, the only way to diagnose trabecular osteoporosis with confidence *before* bone failure has occurred is by iliac crest bone biopsy (see Chapter 6). The mean trabecular bone volume/volume ratio in young adults is 26 percent with a range of 17 to 35 percent. There is a rapid loss of trabecular bone in middle life (Fig. 2-15), and nearly half the elderly population have values below 17 percent, i.e., trabecular osteoporosis. Patients with two or more compressed vertebra generally have trabecular bone volumes below 12 percent and suffer from accelerated trabecular osteoporosis (Fig. 2-16).

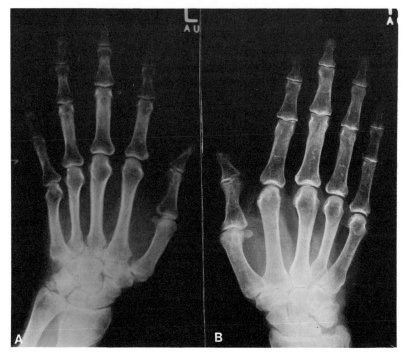

Fig. 2-13. Hand x-rays from a case of mild osteoporosis with normal metacarpal cortical width (A) and a case of severe osteoporosis with greatly reduced cortical width (B).

SEQUENTIAL OBSERVATIONS

In the treatment of osteoporosis, all that the practicing clinician can hope to achieve at present is the prevention of further bone loss, or at best a small positive bone balance. Clearly, compressed vertebrae will not re-expand, and every further compression in a patient established on therapy must be regarded as a therapeutic failure. It is therefore essential that the spinal radiographs should be repeated and examined carefully at least once a year, and the therapy modified if significant deterioration occurs. Continuing loss of bone can, however, be monitored more sensitively by repeating the hand x-rays annually and measuring cortical width very precisely (with needle calipers) at the midpoints of the second, third and fourth metacarpals of each hand. If these measurements are performed in duplicate, the mean value has

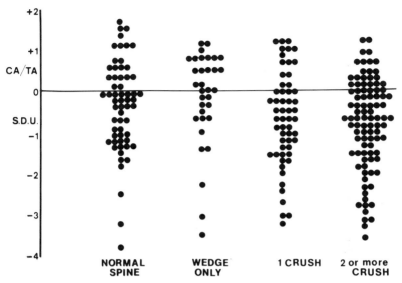

Fig. 2-14. Metacarpal cortical-area/total-area ratios in postmenopausal women with varying degrees of spinal osteoporosis, expressed as standard deviations from the normal mean for age and sex. Note the progressive downward displacement of the data with deterioration of the spine, but note also that most of the individual values fall within the normal range for age.

an error of less than 1 percent, and the technique will detect continuing bone loss after a period of about one year. For this technique to be successful, great care should be taken to eliminate magnification errors by ensuring that the hands are fully in contact with the x-ray cassette when the radiographs are taken.

The spinal densitometric techniques mentioned above are more sensitive, though probably less precise. With the best techniques available, vertebral bone loss is detectable within six months.

BIOCHEMICAL DIAGNOSIS

Osteoporosis is a *state* of bone that produces no specific biochemical signal, but the *process* that leads to the osteoporotic state produces various biochemical abnormalities. It is therefore possible to recognize the preosteoporotic, bone-losing state whether or not the patient is os-

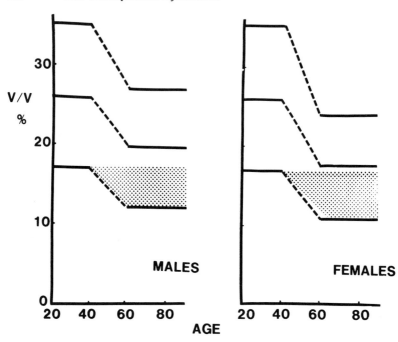

Fig. 2-15. Diagrammatic representation of the change in iliac crest trabecular bone volume with age in males and females. The stippled area represents the fraction of the normal population who fall below the young normal lower limit.

teoporotic at the time of observation. The bone-losing state can be recognized in the following ways:

1. *Fasting urine calcium.* A high fasting urinary calcium/creatinine ratio (upper normal limit about 0.4 mmol/mmol) generally indicates a negative calcium balance, whether this is due to a high rate of bone resorption or a low rate of bone formation. The converse does not hold good, however. In severe calcium malabsorption negative calcium balance may be present when the fasting urinary calcium is in the normal range.

2. *Fasting urine hydroxyproline.* A raised fasting urinary hydroxyproline creatinine ratio (upper normal limit about 0.017 mmol/mmol) indicates an increased rate of bone resorption and generally indicates negative bone balance. However, if bone formation rate is also high, as in Paget's disease and hyperthyroidism, the bone balance may be zero.

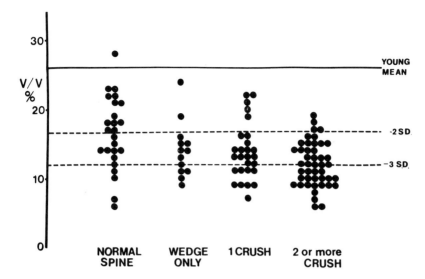

Fig. 2-16. Iliac crest trabecular bone volumes in postmenopausal women with varying degrees of spinal osteoporosis. Note that virtually all crush fracture patients fall below the young normal lower limit and about half of them fall below the lower limit for their age.

3. *Plasma alkaline phosphatase.* In most subjects who are losing bone and developing osteoporosis, the plasma alkaline phosphatase is in the high normal range, but really high values suggest osteomalacia, Paget's disease, or some other bone condition, unless of course they are due to liver disease. The plasma alkaline phosphatase is therefore most useful in the sense that a value in the low normal range makes rapid bone loss very unlikely. (There is no really satisfactory routine procedure for separating the bone and nonbone phosphatases, but the former is more heat-labile than the latter and the "heat stability index" is sometimes of assistance.)

DISTINCTION BETWEEN OSTEOMALACIA AND OSTEOPOROSIS

Confusion between osteomalacia and osteoporosis should seldom arise, although it is of course possible for the two conditions to coexist. It is extremely unusual for pure osteomalacia to present with compression fractures of the vertebrae, and it is rare to find osteomalacia in a patient presenting with spinal osteoporosis. Osteomalacic vertebrae may look normal or increased in "density." If biconcavity is present, it is extremely uniform and regular. Cortical width in the peripheral bones is markedly reduced and they may show pseudofractures. The plasma alkaline phosphatase is raised above the normal range, which is rare in osteoporosis except after a fracture episode. The plasma calcium and phosphate levels are generally low. Above all, the urine calcium is very low in most forms of osteomalacia, whereas it is normal or high in osteoporosis. In the three main osteoporotic fracture groups (wrist, spine, and femoral neck) it is only in the femoral neck cases, and then only in the oldest subjects, that there is a significant prevalence of osteomalacia.

PREVALENCE

The Effect of Age

Simple Osteoporosis

All vertebrate mammals lose bone with age. In the human species, loss of bone starts at or about the time of the menopause in women and perhaps somewhat later in men. Cortical bone loss continues to the end of life in both sexes at a rate of about 1 percent per annum in women and 0.5 percent per annum in men. The result is that an increasing proportion of the population develop cortical osteoporosis with advancing age. In women, 50 percent have cortical osteoporosis by age 70 and 100 percent by age 90. In men, 50 percent have cortical osteoporosis by the age of 80 (Fig. 2-12).

Trabecular bone behaves rather differently. Women begin to lose vertebral bone within the third and fourth decades of life. There is a substantial loss in middle life in both sexes, but a new equilibrium is established at about the age of 60, after which there is very little further loss in the normal population. The mean trabecular volume/volume ratio is about 17 percent from the age of 60 onwards (slightly higher in men than women), with the result that 40 percent of women and a rather smaller proportion of men over the age of 60 suffer from trabecular osteoporosis (Fig. 2-15).

It has already been indicated that a distinction needs to be made between subjects with a degree of osteoporosis that is "normal" for their age (simple osteoporosis) and those with a degree that is greater than would be expected for their age (accelerated osteoporosis). This distinction can often (but not always) be made on spinal radiographs, because it is only the cases of two or more compression fractures in whom the osteoporosis is consistently of the accelerated type; the presence of wedged vertebrae or even one crushed vertebra must not be taken to indicate a more severe degree of osteoporosis than is compatible with normal aging (Fig. 2-6). This is important because no "cause" for the osteoporosis other than aging is likely to be found in the patients with simple osteoporosis.

BONE FORMATION AND RESORPTION

It is axiomatic that a reduction in bone mass must be due to a decline in bone formation, an increase in bone resorption, or a combination of the two. Very little is known about the dynamics of the process responsible for cortical bone loss, but a substantial amount of information is available about trabecular bone loss because of the widespread practice of bone biopsy.

Figure 2-17 illustrates the trabecular volume/volume ratios in young normal, old normal, and osteoporotic men and women. It will be seen that there is a very significant reduction in bone volume with age in both sexes and a further reduction in crush fracture cases in both sexes, as was implied above. The immediate causes of these changes are illustrated in Figures 2-18 and 2-19.

Figure 2-18 shows the extent of the forming surfaces (determined by histomorphometry) in the three male and female groups. Forming surfaces do not change with age in normal women, but are slightly lower in osteoporotic than in normal elderly women. In the men, on the other hand, there is a very significant decline in forming surfaces with age but little difference between normal and osteoporotic elderly men. Thus it seems unlikely that a fall in bone formation is responsible for simple osteoporosis in women, although it may be contributory to accelerated osteoporosis. In men, on the other hand, it is likely that a decline in bone formation accounts for simple osteoporosis but makes no further contribution to accelerated osteoporosis.

The corresponding surface resorption data are shown in Figure 2-19. Percentage surface resorption is significantly higher in old women than in young women, and significantly higher again in osteoporotic

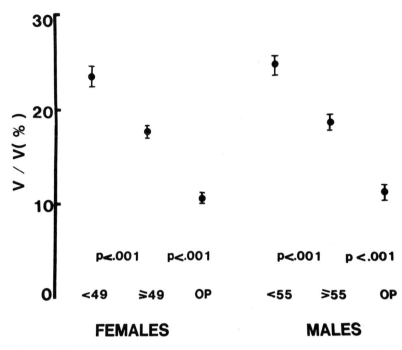

Fig. 2-17. Mean trabecular bone volumes ($\pm$ standard error) in young and old normal and osteoporotic men and women.

than normal elderly women. It does not rise with age in normal men but is significantly raised in men with accelerated osteoporosis. The data can be summarized as follows: In men, simple osteoporosis is due to reduced bone formation and accelerated osteoporosis to the addition of increased resorption. In women, simple osteoporosis is due to increased resorption and accelerated osteoporosis to a further increase in resorption with some decline in formation.

FRACTURES IN THE ELDERLY

The principal fractures associated with osteoporosis are those of the distal forearm, the vertebrae, and the femoral neck. (The details regarding the epidemiology of all age-related fractures are presented in Chapter 3.) There is a steep rise in the distal forearm fracture rate in

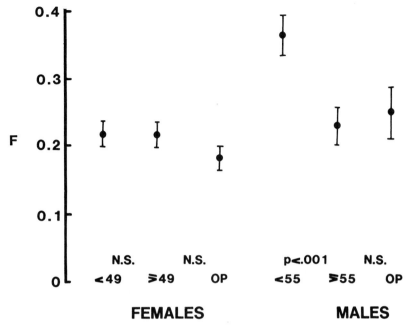

Fig. 2-18.   Mean forming surfaces (intercepts per microscopic field) in the same cases as Figure 2-17. Note that there is little change in forming surfaces in women but a large fall with age in men.

women from about the time of menopause, but little change with age in men. In fact, the fracture is for all intents and purposes a fracture of postmenopausal women. Forearm densitometry has shown significantly less bone in wrist fracture cases than in age-matched controls, although the bone deficit is only about 10 percent. It may be that the trauma involved in falling on the outstretched arm (which is the cause of this fracture) is so severe that only a small bone deficit is required to cause critical weakness of the bone. It is of considerable interest that the Singh index (which is a subjective but nonetheless useful indicator of trabecular bone status in the proximal femur) may also be significantly lower in wrist fracture cases than age-matched controls (Fig. 2-8). The vertebral crush fractures have been discussed above and are undoubtedly a manifestation of trabecular bone loss. Wedging of the vertebrae is present in about 60 percent of elderly women, but only 5 to 10 percent develop two or more crush fractures. In these patients, the Singh

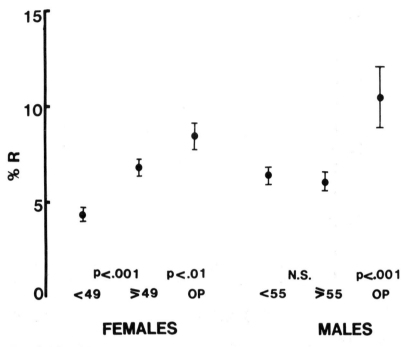

Fig. 2-19. Mean percent surface resorption in iliac crest samples from the same cases as Figures 2-17 and 2-18. Note the rise in resorption with age in women, and the further rise in osteoporotics of both sexes.

index is significantly reduced, as also is cortical bone status, though to a lesser degree (Figs. 2-9 and 2-14).

Femoral neck fractures are more complex. There has been considerable uncertainty as to whether this should be regarded as a cortical or trabecular bone fracture, whether it can be entirely accounted for by loss of bone, and whether the bone status of fracture cases differs from that of age-matched controls. These questions can now be answered. The rise in femoral neck fractures with age in both sexes is steeper than can be accounted for by loss of bone alone; an important contributory factor is the increasing incidence of falls with advancing age, particularly in women, due to the increasing prevalence of cardiovascular and cerebrovascular disease with age, to impaired vision and to other disabilities associated with aging. Nonetheless, falls alone do not explain the fractures; loss of bone is a vital contributory cause. Not only do the

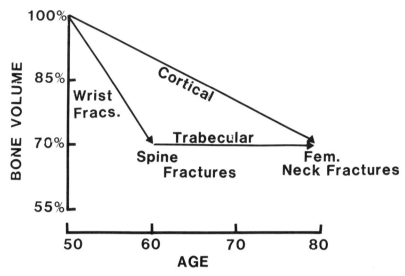

Fig. 2-20. Diagrammatic representation of the relation between bone loss and fractures. Wrist and spine fractures are associated with loss of trabecular bone. Femoral neck fractures occur when cortical loss "catches up" with trabecular loss.

fracture cases suffer from cortical and trabecular osteoporosis (as would of course be expected from their age), but as a group they are significantly more osteoporotic than age-matched controls in respect of both trabecular and cortical bone. However, the discrimination between fracture cases and controls is most significant when *both* a cortical bone measurement (such as the metacarpal CA/TA) and a trabecular bone measurement (such as the Singh index) are taken into account. This means that fracture risk is a function of the degree of osteoporosis; the patients with the most severe loss of bone are the ones most liable to fracture, and fracture cases as a group therefore show significantly poorer bone status than age-matched controls. The simplest way to understand these fractures is illustrated in Figure 2-20. The wrist fractures occur during the phase of rapid trabecular bone loss, the spine fractures when exceptional trabecular bone loss has occurred, and the femoral neck fractures when the cortical bone loss has caught up with the trabecular bone loss.

All these three fractures are inter-related, i.e., the patients who

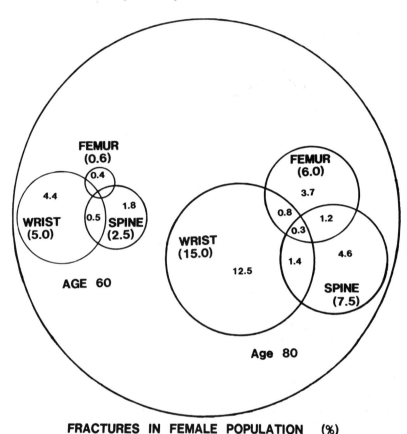

FRACTURES IN FEMALE POPULATION   (%)

Fig. 2-21. Diagrammatic representation of fracture prevalence in women by age 60 and age 80. The outer circle represents the whole population. The inner circles represent the fracture populations drawn to scale. The overlapping areas represent cases with more than one fracture. The numbers denote the percentages of the total population who have sustained the different fractures.

have had a wrist fracture incur a significantly increased risk of vertebral and/or femoral neck fracture, patients with vertebral fractures are at increased risk for wrist and femoral neck fractures, and patients with femoral neck fractures have had significantly more wrist fractures and vertebral fractures than age-matched controls. The cumulative prevalence of all these fractures in women is about 7 percent by age 60 and about 25 percent by age 80 (Fig. 2-21).

PATHOGENESIS

Primary Osteoporosis

The term osteoporosis implies that the condition is not associated with any of the diseases or disorders that are known to produce an osteoporotic state, notably, hyperthyroidism, Cushing's syndrome, and corticosteroid therapy. It should not be taken to imply that no risk factors have been identified, but simply that a recognized casual condition has not been established. Primary osteoporosis may be simple or accelerated.

Simple Primary Osteoporosis

Simple primary osteoporosis in women is the result of the increased bone resorption associated with the menopause. Estrogenic hormones tend to protect the bone against the resorbing action of parathyroid hormone. The decline in estrogen levels at the menopause is associated with a rise in bone resorption attributable to the increased sensitivity of the bone to these bone-resorbing agents. It is possible that this estrogen effect is mediated through calcitonin, since calcitonin levels are low in menopausal females and blood calcitonin rises during estrogen therapy. Whether the action of estrogens on bone is direct or indirect, this general concept of the pathogenesis of postmenopausal osteoporosis remains the same. The menopausal increase in bone resorption is associated with small but significant rises in the fasting plasma calcium, phosphate and alkaline phosphatase levels, and in urinary calcium and hydroxyproline excretion. There may also be a small decline in calcium absorption, possibly mediated through a decline in the plasma level of the biologically active forms of vitamin $D_3, 1,25(OH)_2D_3$, but this is currently debatable.

The cause of the decline in bone formation with age that results in simple osteoporosis in the male sex is unknown at the present time, but it may reflect a decline in testicular and/or adrenal androgen production. There is no clear rise in urinary calcium or hydroxyproline with age in men, nor has any change in plasma calcium or alkaline phosphatase levels been reported. There is, however, a decline in skinfold thickness from about the age of 55 onwards, which may also reflect a decline in androgen levels.

Accelerated Osteoporosis

The principal metabolic abnormality that has been defined in men and women with vertebral compression fractures (accelerated osteoporosis) is malabsorption of calcium, which is present in a high proportion of these cases. The cause of this malabsorption is uncertain. It has been suggested that it is due to a deficiency of $1,25(OH)_2D_3$ due to a functional depression of 1α-hydroxylase, but there is no agreement on this point and an alternative explanation might be that these patients (or some of them) are suffering from an end-organ failure in the gastrointestinal tract.

The hormonal status of osteoporotic patients is more controversial. In postmenopausal women an inverse relationship between plasma estrogen levels and fasting urinary calcium has been reported by several different groups. It would imply that bone resorption is more rapid in the patients with the lowest estrogen levels, but hormone assays in age-matched osteoporotic and normal postmenopausal women have yielded conflicting and equivocal results. There are also reports of increments in parathyroid hormone in aging osteoporotic females that may reflect prolonged subclinical calcium deficient states due to poor dietary habits. In males, there is no doubt that true hypogonadism is associated with osteoporosis (possibly due to reduced bone formation), but in the majority of osteoporotic male subjects plasma testosterone levels are within the normal range.

There are several other risk factors that probably contribute to accelerated osteoporosis in various ways. The best documented of these is alcohol. There is strong evidence that alcoholics are more liable to osteoporosis than the population at large, and a history of high alcohol intake can be obtained from a number of male osteoporotics. The mechanism is obscure. It has been reported that malabsorption of calcium is a feature of these cases and is directly related to the degree of liver damage, which might suggest that the malabsorption is secondary to a deficiency of $25(OH)D_3$ from impaired liver synthesis. If this were the case, however, osteomalacia should also be a feature of alcoholism, but this has not been reported. Perhaps a more likely explanation is that alcoholics drink little milk and are liable to malnutrition of all kinds; dietary calcium deficiency may be the problem.

Gastrointestinal surgery probably constitutes another factor because of the effect of certain bypass operations on calcium absorption. Again this is more likely to be a feature of male than female osteoporotics. Diabetes is probably another risk factor, possibly due to the adverse effect of insulin deficiency on protein synthesis. Case control studies have shown a significant association between diabetes and fractures. However, diabetes is not a common finding in osteoporotic subjects—either male or female.

Another well recognized risk factor is alactasia, which has been reported as present in 30 percent of osteoporotic subjects in several different series. It is not clear whether the connection with osteoporosis is malabsorption of calcium secondary to the bowel defect or the low calcium intake of alactasic subjects. Low calcium intake is of course itself a risk factor for osteoporosis in both males and females, but it cannot often be identified as the only causal factor. High protein intake is known to raise urinary calcium and produce a negative calcium balance, and it might be expected to be a risk factor for osteoporosis. It is possible, however, that calcium requirement is a function of protein intake and that the low fracture rate in developing countries despite low calcium intake reflects low calcium requirements in the presence of low protein intakes.

Liver disease may constitute another risk factor, but the evidence on this point is weak. There is no doubt that osteoporosis (and osteomalacia) are common in primary biliary cirrhosis, in which condition a severe steatorrhoea is associated with malabsorption of calcium and vitamin D. What is far less certain is whether portal cirrhosis is associated with osteoporosis. This calls for further investigation.

SECONDARY OSTEOPOROSIS

Hyperadrenocorticism

Vertebral crush fractures are a well recognized feature of Cushing's disease and are also associated with corticosteroid therapy. It has been thought since the time of Albright that this form of osteoporosis is due to the depression of new bone formation resulting from the effect of corticosteroids on protein synthesis, but although it is true that skinfold thickness is reduced in these patients and that there is some reduction in the appositional growth rate in bone biopsies, increased bone resorption is a more striking feature of these cases than the biopsies from decreased bone formation (Table 2-1). The cause of this increase in bone resorption is not entirely clear, but it may be secondary to inhibi-

Table 2-1
Trabecular bone volume (V), forming surfaces (intercepts per field) (F) and percent resorbing surfaces (R) in normal, thyrotoxic and corticosteroid-treated postmenopausal women (Mean values ± S.E.).

Group	N	V	F	R
Normal (postmortem)	59	17.6 ± 0.59	0.80 ± 0.07	6.81 ± 0.41
Steroid-treated	32	11.4 ± 0.80*	0.71 ± 0.09	9.40 ± 0.72*
Thyrotoxic	10	16.0 ± 1.53	1.40 ± 0.25*	13.40 ± 3.20*

* p 0.001 compared with normal group

tion of calcium absorption by corticosteroids, for which there is a good deal of clinical and experimental evidence. This reduced calcium absorption does not appear to be due to an effect of corticosteroids on vitamin D metabolism, but rather to an end-organ effect in the gastrointestinal tract. It should be emphasized that Cushing's syndrome may be present in elderly women as osteoporosis without any of the physical signs usually associated with glucocorticoid excess.

Hyperthyroidism

Spinal osteoporosis is a well recognized feature of hyperthyroidism, but it is not nearly as common as it used to be when treatment of hyperthyroidism was less effective than it is today. At the histologic level there is a very striking increase in bone resorption, but also a corresponding increase in bone formation with the result that trabecular bone volume is generally normal (Table 2-1). These changes probably reflect a direct effect of thyroid hormone on bone. There is a rise in urinary calcium and hydroxyproline excretion and a significant elevation in plasma alkaline phosphatase. In addition, plasma calcium and phosphate levels tend to be slightly raised. Marginal hypercalcemia tends to reduce parathyroid hormone and $1,25(OH)_2D_3$ levels, resulting in a reduction in calcium absorption. The hyperphosphatemia results from two causes—increased bone resorption and increased tubular reabsorption of phosphate secondary to parathyroid suppression.

Disuse Osteoporosis

The third major cause of secondary osteoporosis is disuse or weightlessness. Once again, it has been classically attributed to reduced new bone formation, since it is well established that mechanical stresses on bone stimulate new bone formation. In reality, however, histologic and kinetic studies have shown a remarkable increase in bone resorption following immobilization, e.g., in neurologic injuries that lead to a rapid loss of trabecular bone in particular. Both mechanical weight bearing and muscle tension appear to be involved in the maintenance of bone health, but the latter factor is probably the more important of the two, inasmuch as osteoporosis may develop rapidly in a limb immobilized in plaster in the absence of any nerve or muscle injury. Why bone resorption should increase in response to weightlessness is quite unknown.

Hyperparathyroidism

Although trabecular osteoporosis is relatively uncommon in hyperparathyroidism (primary or secondary), cortical osteoporosis undoubtedly occurs. Cortical bone loss is accelerated in primary hyperparathyroidism and cross-sectional measurements demonstrate reduced cortical width in these cases, particularly in postmenopausal women. In secondary hyperparathyroidism (osteomalacia and renal failure), the cortical width is significantly reduced and bone loss is accelerated. Why hyperparathyroidism should affect cortical rather than trabecular bone is not known unless the increased osteoid-covered surfaces, which are a feature of hyperparathyroidism, protect trabecular bone (where turnover is high) against resorption but do not protect cortical bone (in which turnover is much lower) in a similar way. The relatively independent behavior of cortical and trabecular bone is nowhere better illustrated than in renal failure, where the vertebral column may show sclerotic changes at the same time as cortical thinning in the peripheral bone is sufficiently severe to give rise to fractures. Vertebral osteoporosis does occur occasionally in primary hyperparathyroidism, but probably no more often than would be expected by chance.

BIBLIOGRAPHY

Barzel U (ed): Osteoporosis. New York: Grune and Stratton, 1979

DeLuca HF, Frost HM, Jee WSS, Johnston CC, Jr, Parfitt AM (eds): Osteoporosis. Baltimore, University Park Press, 1981

Davidson BF, Ross RK, Paganini-Hill A, Hammond GD, Siiteri PK, Judd HL: Total and free estrogens and androgens in postmenopausal women with hip fractures. J Clin Endocrinol Metab 54:115–119, 1982

Fujita T, Okuyama Y, Handa N, Orimo H, Ohata M, Yoshikawa M, Akiyama H, Kogure T: Age dependent bone loss after gastrectomy. J Am Geriatrics Soc 19:840–846, 1971

Insogna KL, Lewis AM, Lipinski BA, Brynat C, Baran DT: Effect of age on serum immuoreactive parathyroid hormone and its biological effects. J Clin Endocrinol Metab 53:1072–1075, 1981

Kleerekoper M, Sudhaker DR, Frame B, LaRocque RD, Feigelman T, Matkovic V, Avioli LU: Occult Cushing's syndrome presenting with osteoporosis. Henry Ford Hosp Med J 28:132–137, 1980

Lund BJ, Sørensen OH, Lund BJ, Agner E: Serum 1,25-Dihydroxyvitamin D in normal subjects and in patients with postmenopausal osteopenia, influence of age, renal function and estrogen therapy. Hormone Metab Res 14:271–274, 1982

Morimoto S, Tsuji M, Okada Y, Onishi T, Kumahara Y: The effect of estrogens on human calcitonin secretion after calcium infusion in elderly female subjects. Clin Endocrinol 13:135–143, 1980

Nordin BEC (ed): Osteoporosis. Clinics in endocrinology and metabolism, 2. London, Saunders, 1973

Riggs BL, Hamstra A, DeLuca HF: Assessment of 25-hydroxyvitamin D 1α-hydroxylase reserve in postmenopausal osteoporosis by administration of parathyroid extract. J Clin Endocrinol Metab 53:833–835, 1981

Riggs BL, Wahner HW, Dunn WL, Mazess RB, Offord KP, Melton LG: Differential changes in bone mineral density of the appendicular and axial skeleton with aging. J Clin Invest 67:328–335, 1981

Smith D, Khairi MRA, Johnston Jr, CC: The loss of bone mineral with aging and its relationship to risk fracture. J Clin Endocrinol Metab 56:311–318, 1975

Slovik DM, Adams JS, New RM, Holick MF, Potts JT: Deficient production of 1,25-dehydroxyvitamin D in elderly osteoporotic patients. N Engl Med 305:372–374, 1981

Sørensen O, Lumholtz B, Lund B, Lund B, Hjelmstrand I, Mosekilde L, Melsen F, Bishop J, Norman A: Acute effects of parathyroid hormone on vitamin D metabolism in patients with the bone loss of aging. J Clin Endocrinol Metab 54:1258–1261, 1982

Stevenson J, Abeyasekera G, Hillyard C, Phang KG, MacIntyre I, Campbell S, Townsend P, Young O, Whitehead M: Calcitonin and the calcium regulating hormones in postmenopausal women: Effect of estrogens. Lancet 1:693–695, 1981

Wiske PS, Epstein S, Bell N, Queener S, Edmondson J, Johnston Jr, C: Increases in immunoreactive parathyroid hormone with age. N Eng J Med 300:1419–1421, 1979

3

Epidemiology of Age-related Fractures

L. Joseph Melton, III
B. Lawrence Riggs

WHY STUDY FRACTURE EPIDEMIOLOGY?

Practitioners develop a concept of age-related fractures that is based on the care of individual patients. The study of fractures as they occur in entire populations of people (epidemiology) provides a very different perspective. For example, the overview provided by epidemiology more accurately reflects the impact of osteoporosis and its attendant fractures on society as a whole. By determining the circumstances under which such fractures are common in the population, epidemiologic investigations can characterize the subgroups at particularly high or very low risk. This information can then be used to design prevention programs or for generation of hypotheses to be tested in subsequent clinical research. Moreover, accurate knowledge of the true clinical spectrum of age-related fractures in the population provides the best information about prognosis and other aspects of the natural history of these disorders and thus may be of assistance in optimal patient management. Although a great deal remains to be learned about the epidemiology of age-related fractures, especially in accurately identifying risk factors, the picture is becoming clearer. The knowledge that we have acquired to date on this fascinating subject is presented here to provide a context for the more detailed discussions of pathophysiology and treatment in subsequent chapters.

45

THE MAGNITUDE OF THE PROBLEM

Fractures are quite common, especially among the young and the very old. Figure 3-1 shows the typical biphasic pattern for limb fractures that is characteristic of the general distribution of fractures as a function of age. The location of the fractures and their relationship to antecedent trauma are quite dissimilar in the two extremes of age. This chapter is most concerned with fractures among older persons because these fractures are the most likely to be associated with osteoporosis. Traditionally, fractures of the vertebrae, distal forearm, and proximal femur among elderly persons, especially when they occur in association with only minimal or moderate trauma, have been considered to be due to osteoporosis. Recent detailed studies have revealed, however, that fractures of the proximal humerus and most pelvic fractures should definitely be included in this category and that the risk of most other limb fractures increases with advancing age as well (Table 3-1). Indeed, half or more of all fractures among adults may be related to osteoporosis. The cumulative lifetime risk of having an age-related fracture is substantial, as shown in Figure 3-2. Up to 33 percent of women and more than 17 percent of men could experience a hip fracture by age 90. The proportions of women and men who could have a Colles fracture as an adult are about 24 percent and 5 percent, respectively. For fractures of the proximal humerus, the respective figures are 12 percent and 4 percent, and for pelvic fractures, they are 9 percent and 2.5 percent. Accurate data on the cumulative incidence of vertebral fractures are not available, but the prevalence of such fractures among 70-year-old Danish women was reported to be 21 percent. Thus, most practitioners will be faced with the task of managing patients with one or more age-related fractures.

The public health impact of age-related fractures can be measured in terms of mortality and morbidity as well. Hip fractures are by far the most serious, of course, and cause a 12 percent reduction in expected survival rates. The increased mortality occurs primarily in the first four months after the hip fracture. Although subsequent survival is generally poor for these usually elderly patients, it is no less than expected for persons of comparable age and sex in the general population. Because hip fractures are so common, they are an important cause of death and are largely responsible for the observation that falls are the leading cause of accidental death among men and women older than age 75 in the United States and the second leading cause among those age

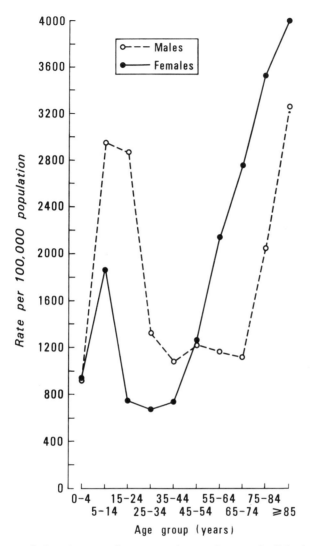

Fig. 3-1. Age- and sex-specific incidence of all limb fractures among the residents of Rochester, Minnesota, 1969–1971. (From Garraway WM, Stauffer RN, Kurland LT, O'Fallon WM: Limb fractures in a defined population. I. Frequency and distribution. Mayo Clin Proc 54:701–707, 1979. Reproduced with permission of the author and publisher.)

Table 3-1
Estimated excess fractures among United States whites age 40 or older in 1975, based on fracture rates among those age 30 to 39*

| Fracture sites | Number of fractures | | | % of total for each site |
	Observed in those ≥40 yr old	Expected at 30–39 yr old rates	Excess	
MEN				
Proximal femur	35,654	2,771	32,883	92.2
Proximal humerus	18,542	9,255	9,287	50.1
Distal forearm	62,487	58,616	3,871	6.2
Pelvis	10,977	1,851	9,126	83.1
All other limb fractures	253,362	271,482	0	0
Subtotal	381,022		55,167	14.5
WOMEN				
Proximal femur	156,680	2,238	154,442	98.6
Proximal humerus	65,733	4,483	61,250	93.2
Distal forearm	205,391	29,888	175,503	85.4
Pelvis	33,621	8,966	24,655	73.3
All other limb fractures	317,580	198,007	119,573	37.7
Subtotal	779,005		535,423	68.7
All sites, both sexes	1,160,027 per year		590,590	50.9
				per year

*Age- and sex-specific fracture rates are from the population of Rochester, Minnesota.

45 to 74. Other fractures result in death less often except when the patient has substantial associated injuries, as is often the case with pelvic fractures due to severe trauma, for example. Death is not the only adverse outcome either. Rehabilitation is often unsuccessful among the elderly patients. At least half of those who could walk before sustaining a hip fracture cannot walk subsequently. The ability of such patients to get about and care for themselves is greatly compromised, and their

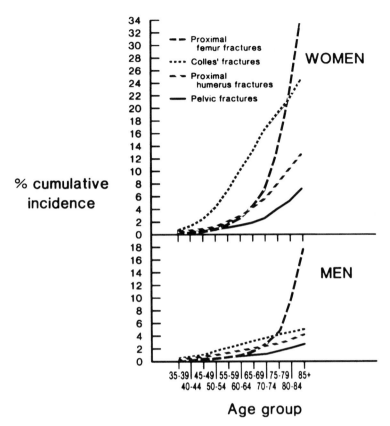

Fig. 3-2. Cumulative incidence of various age-related fractures over a lifetime for men and women residents of Rochester, Minnesota.

quality of life is considerably reduced. As many as half of all patients with hip fracture are unable to live independently after the fracture and must be cared for in a nursing home.

The economic burden of age-related fractures is truly enormous because of the large number of people involved and the expensive and protracted care that is often required. About a fourth of all patients with limb fractures require hospitalization, and the mean hospital stay increases from 13.6 days among those age 25 to 44, to 32.6 days among those older than age 65. Fractures of the proximal femur account for more than half of all days of hospitalization for limb fractures. The cost of the acute care alone for fractures of the proximal femur has been estimated to exceed one billion dollars annually in the United States. The cost of acute care for Colles' fractures in adults may reach 140 million dollars each year. The costs for fractures at the other sites, such as vertebrae and proximal humerus, have apparently not been determined, nor have the costs for rehabilitation and long-term institutionalization for any of these fracture sites. Such expenses are undoubtedly substantial and impose a formidable burden on the entire medical-care system. These costs will increase as the number of elderly people grows, both in absolute terms and as a proportion of the total population.

PRINCIPLES OF METHODOLOGY

Several methodologic problems inherent in the study of age-related fractures should be recognized. The most useful tool for studying the occurrence of fractures, identifying high-risk groups, and measuring differences between populations is the incidence rate. For determining the incidence of a particular fracture, all new cases that occur in some circumscribed population during a specified period must be identified. In the typical clinical study, some new cases are identified but the population from which the cases originated cannot be precisely described, a factor that precludes accurate calculation of an incidence *rate*.

$$\text{Incidence rate per } 100{,}000 \text{ person-years} = \frac{\text{number of new fracture cases during a specified period}}{\text{person-years at risk during the same period}} \times 100{,}000$$

Some authors have quoted the *ratio* of fracture cases to all hospital admissions, but this quantity cannot be used to study occurrence of fractures in the population. In a strict sense, the incidence rate refers to the occurrence of fractures among those at risk. Thus the ideal study would describe the incidence of age-related fractures among those in the population with osteoporosis. Because this information is rarely available, incidence rates are usually calculated for the entire population with the implied assumption that everyone is at risk.

In other instances, the denominator (the population of a city or county for which census data exist) may be known, but the exact number of new cases cannot be determined. This may result from inability to canvass all medical-care providers for new fracture cases or from inherent difficulty in finding new cases. Identification of new hip fractures is relatively easy because patients seek medical care and are usually hospitalized. In contrast, patients with Colles' fractures are usually seen as outpatients and are treated by a much wider variety of practitioners, and patients with vertebral fractures may not seek medical care at all. These observations are reflected in the literature, where epidemiologic studies of hip fracture predominate. The incidence of vertebral fractures is essentially unknown because ascertainment of cases has proved to be such a formidable problem.

If the incidence of a particular fracture cannot be determined, it may still be possible to define its prevalence—i.e., the proportion of persons in a population at some specific time who have the fracture or have a history of the fracture.

$$\text{Prevalence rate per 100,000 population} = \frac{\text{number of persons with history of fracture at a specified time}}{\text{population at risk at the same time}} \times 100,000$$

The prevalence rate has value as an indicator of the magnitude of the burden imposed by such patients in the community, but it is often inappropriately used in place of incidence data. Prevalence and incidence are related (prevalence equals incidence multiplied by duration of disease); but because prevalence rates are affected by survival, migration, and other factors, they are usually very unreliable estimators of incidence.

Additional problems are encountered when the epidemiologic features of fractures in two different populations are compared. For example, overall incidence rates would appear to be unequal if one group had disproportionately more elderly women, even if the incidence rates in each sex and age group were identical for the two populations. For derivation of a fair comparison, the rates must be adjusted. This modification is usually accomplished by applying the rates for each age and sex (age- and sex-specific incidence rates) to the number of persons in each comparable group in some standard population and determining the resultant number of cases under such conditions. The estimated number of cases is then divided by the total standard population and multiplied by a standard factor—such as 100,000—to arrive at a new "adjusted" incidence rate. The standard used here is the structure of the United States white population in 1970. It is very important to note that age and sex adjustment does not correct for differences in the clinical spectrum of fracture cases in various groups. The true clinical spectrum of any given fracture is reflected by the incidence cases because they represent all occurrences in the population under study. The prevalence cases represent the survivors, who may have very different characteristics. The apparent clinical spectrum of an "unselected" patient series at a medical center is more distorted yet because the cases may be a mixture of new and old, and because referral patterns impose intense patient selection even if the investigators do not.

Further difficulties arise when one moves beyond descriptive studies of fractures to investigations of etiologic factors. Determining the characteristics of the cases is relatively easy, although the advanced age of many patients makes some kinds of data difficult to obtain. It is much harder to decide whether these characteristics are different from those expected. A variety of chronic diseases and abnormal physiologic states could be attributed simply to the fact that most of the patients are elderly. Thus, appropriate control groups from the general population are needed for comparison. Hospital or referral center control subjects are rarely representative of the general population. Merely describing the differences in the proportion of cases and control subjects who have each supposed risk factor is insufficient. For assessment of the degree of risk associated with any particular factor in a case-control study, it is necessary to calculate an odds ratio, which is typically in the following form:

$$\text{Odds ratio} = \frac{\text{(number of fracture cases with the factor)}}{\text{(number of fracture cases without the factor)}} \quad \frac{\text{(number of controls without the factor)}}{\text{(number of controls with the factor)}}$$

The odds ratio is an estimate of the relative risk, which can be obtained directly from a prospective cohort study:

$$\text{Relative risk} = \frac{\text{incidence of fractures among those exposed to the factor}}{\text{incidence of fractures among those unexposed to the factor}}$$

Very few cohort studies, other than clinical trials, have been undertaken to analyze fracture risk factors. Case-control studies are only slightly more common.

Because of the aforementioned problems, the epidemiologic features of age-related fractures have been studied in relatively few settings. Most investigations have been undertaken where medical care is under centralized control—e.g., in Scandinavia and certain other European countries—although special surveys have been conducted in many regions. Despite the magnitude of the problem of age-related fractures in the United States, few population-based studies have been conducted except in the unique community of Rochester, Minnesota. Because much of the data to be described was derived from Rochester, a brief description of the situation in that community is warranted. The population of Rochester is isolated from other large urban centers, and medical care for the residents is concentrated among relatively few providers. The largest of these is the Mayo Clinic, which provides about 80 percent of the care. Each of the providers uses a unit record system in which all of a person's medical data, both inpatient and outpatient, is contained in a single dossier. Moreover, an index to the unit records of each provider has been developed by the Mayo Clinic and the Rochester Epidemiology Program Project. Thus, all Rochester residents in whom a particular fracture has been diagnosed can be identified, and their original medical records can be retrieved and reviewed. This system allows complete case ascertainment in the community and is the key to the accurate population-based studies that have been conducted to date. The complete community coverage also allows the identification of control subjects from the general population.

WHO GETS AGE-RELATED FRACTURES?

Overview of Risk Factors

It is generally conceded that the risk of fracture with any given degree of trauma increases as bone density decreases, although this relationship may not be entirely linear. Conversely, with any given level of bone density, the risk of fracture increases with the amount of force applied by the trauma. There is no convincing evidence that elderly persons have increased fragility of bone independent of that due to age-related bone loss. Thus, the risk of age-related fractures can be expressed as follows:

$$\text{Risk of fracture} = \frac{\text{degree of trauma}}{\text{bone density level}}$$

The risk factors for age-related fractures, then, can be arbitrarily divided into two kinds: (1) those that increase the risk of trauma, in terms of severity, frequency, or both; and (2) those that cause a reduction in bone density. Some factors, such as the hemiplegia that frequently follows a stroke, may do both. The following discussion examines the role of age, sex, geography, and race, along with more specific risk factors for diminished bone density and particular types of trauma.

Age and Sex

Fractures among children and young adults are related to substantial trauma, are somewhat more common in males than in females, and usually involve the shaft of the long bones of the extremities, which consist primarily of cortical bone. An exception is the increased incidence of Colles' fracture in children, which is associated with falls on the outstretched hand and occurs at the epiphysis of the radius. In contrast, the fractures that are related to advanced age, and by extension to osteoporosis, share three distinctive features: (1) the incidence rates are greater among women than among men, (2) the rates increase dramatically with age, and (3) the fractures occur at sites containing large proportions of trabecular bone. These features for some of the most important age-related fracture sites are shown in Figure 3-3.

The classic example of age-related fractures is fracture of the proximal femur. The incidence among women rises exponentially from 9 per 100,000 person-years for age 35 to 44, to a peak rate of 3,317 per 100,000 person-years (or 3.3 percent per year) for women age 85 or older. The incidence among men age 35 to 44 is similar to that for women, 10 per 100,000 person-years, but the peak reached among those age 85 or older, 1,833 per 100,000 person-years, is only half as great. Incidence rates for women are substantially greater than those for men at all ages beyond 50. Overall, about 98 percent of all fractures of the proximal femur occur among persons age 35 or older, and more than 80 percent occur in women. Incidence rates for the two major types of hip fracture, cervical and intertrochanteric, are similar for each age and sex group in Rochester except for the suggestion of a somewhat more rapid increase in incidence of intertrochanteric fractures in the ninth decade of life. Other investigators have reported an excess of either cervical or intertrochanteric fractures.

A similar pattern of age- and sex-specific incidence among women can be noted for fractures of the proximal humerus and of the pelvis

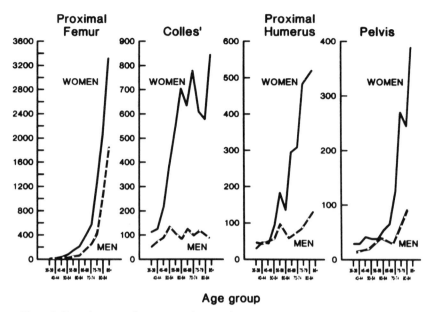

Fig. 3-3. Age- and sex-specific incidence rates per 100,000 person-years among residents of Rochester, Minnesota, for four age-related fracture sites. (Note that the vertical scale varies for each fracture site.)

(Fig. 3-3). Among men, the incidence of fractures at these two sites does not appear to increase as rapidly with advancing age as in the case of fracture of the proximal femur. About one-third of the fractures of the proximal humerus involve the greater tuberosity, and two-thirds do not. The incidence of fractures involving the greater tuberosity increases with aging but not to the degree seen for the proximal fractures that do not involve the greater tuberosity. This finding may be related to weaker rotator cuff musculature among elderly persons or to a reduced tendency to tense the shoulder muscles to break a fall. On the other hand, most pelvic fractures manifest as either fractures of isolated bones or single breaks in the pelvic ring. The pelvic rami, which contain considerable amounts of trabecular bone, are most commonly involved among elderly patients. Multiple, severe fractures of the pelvis almost always are associated with substantial trauma and usually occur among the young.

Both fractures of the proximal humerus and fractures of the pelvis are common, especially among women. Fractures of the proximal hu-

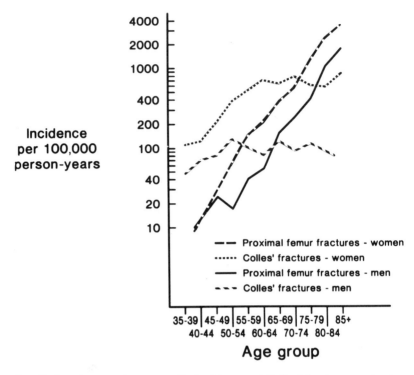

Incidence per 100,000 person-years

- — Proximal femur fractures - women
- ····· Colles' fractures - women
- —— Proximal femur fractures - men
- - - - Colles' fractures - men

35-39 | 45-49 | 55-59 | 65-69 | 75-79 | 85+
40-44 50-54 60-64 70-74 80-84

Age group

Fig. 3-4. Age- and sex-specific incidence of Colles' fracture contrasted with that for hip fracture among residents of Rochester, Minnesota.

merus occur at about 70 percent of the age-adjusted rate for hip fractures when all ages are considered, and pelvic fractures occur at about a third of the rate for hip fractures. The pattern of age- and sex-specific incidence rates for fractures of the proximal femur and of the proximal humerus had been demonstrated in earlier studies of Western populations. The only previous population-based study of pelvic fractures, in the United Kingdom, failed to show a substantial female excess in incidence and also appeared to underestimate the effect of age. These results may have been due to incomplete case ascertainment, inasmuch as age-adjusted rates in the Rochester, Minnesota, study were three times greater for men and eight times greater for women. As already noted, the incidence of vertebral fractures is unknown.

In comparison with other types of age-related fractures, Colles' fractures display a somewhat different pattern of incidence. As shown in Figure 3-3, a substantial excess has been noted among women, as for the other sites, but the steep rise in incidence begins at a much earlier age. Instead of continuing to increase exponentially with age, however, the incidence rates plateau after about age 60. Incidence rates among men show little tendency to rise after age 50. From the epidemiologic standpoint, these differences in the pattern of incidence rates by age and sex may prove to be of greater interest than the overall similarities. In Figure 3-4, the incidence rates for fractures of the proximal femur and for Colles' fractures are replotted on a semilogarithmic grid to emphasize the rate of change in incidence as age increases. It can be seen that the incidence rates for women begin to increase rapidly in the postmenopausal years for both fractures, but the rates for men show a similar tendency. For both men and women, the incidence of fractures of the proximal femur continues to rise rapidly with advancing age thereafter, but this pattern is not maintained for Colles' fractures. These observations provide sufficient evidence to discount any simplistic view of age-related fractures as solely due to the effects of menopause on the bone density of middle-aged women and to the effects of senile osteoporosis among elderly persons of both sexes. More detailed information on the possible mechanisms whereby age (present chapter) and sex (Chapter 5) affect bone density is provided elsewhere in this book.

Geography and Race

The apparent frequency with which age-related fractures occur in different geographic areas varies enormously (see Table 3-2). Some of these geographic differences may be due to methodologic problems such as noncomparable definitions and incomplete case ascertainment. Nevertheless, much of the variation may be real and may provide clues to the etiology of age-related fractures. Claims that some of the apparent geographic differences are due to increasing incidence rates of fractures in recent decades have not been substantiated in Rochester, Minnesota, where incidence rates for both proximal femur and Colles' fractures have been stable for 30 years.

Fracture rates seem to be higher in the temperate zones than in the tropics. Rochester, Minnesota, for example, has the highest reported incidence of hip fractures in the world. This finding does not appear to be due to the direct effect of severe winters, because most hip fractures occur indoors. Moreover, although 40 percent of all limb fractures in Rochester during a recent three-year period were due to falls, less than 8 percent of these falls were on icy or snowy surfaces. An alternative

Table 3-2

Age-adjusted incidence rates per 100,000 person-years for various limb fracture sites in different population groups among persons 35 years of age or older.*

Geographic locality	Proximal femur		Distal forearm or Colles		Proximal humerus	
	Women	Men	Women	Men	Women	Men
USA, Rochester	295.0	126.9	396.4	86.0	78.9	23.3
Sweden, Malmo	203.2	88.3	332.1	49.5	71.5	30.9
New Zealand						
Whites	178.3	80.9				
Maori	88.3	70.9				
Israel, Jerusalem						
American/European-born	174.6	97.2				
Native-born	145.8	92.5				
Asian/African-born	126.4	98.4				
United Kingdom, Oxford/Dundee	114.9	59.2	304.4	72.9	30.2	16.1
Finland	114.1	64.4				
South Africa, Johannesburg						
Whites	217.3	83.2				
Bantu	12.4	12.6				

58

Singapore				
Indian	268.0	117.7	58.3	61.6
Chinese	50.3	90.9		
Malay	20.3	33.0		
Hong Kong	72.4	63.4		
Yugoslavia				
High calcium area	39.7	42.3	221.3	98.1
Low calcium area	91.5	88.4	196.9	112.2

*Age-adjusted to total 1970 United States whites.

suggestion is that fracture rates may vary with latitude as a consequence of different ambient levels of ultraviolet radiation. The number of hospital dismissals for hip fracture, as estimated by the Public Health Service, is lower for the southern region than for the north central region of the United States. The ratio of the number of dismissals observed for the South and the number expected by using Rochester, Minnesota, age- and sex-specific incidence rates of hip fractures, is 1.0, however; an indication that the Rochester rates accurately predict the number of hospital dismissals in the South. The ratio of observed to expected hospital dismissals for hip fracture for the north central region was 1.1 when Rochester rates were used. These data provide no evidence for a gradient of risk with latitude, although the comparison of north central with southern regions in the United States may be too crude to detect subtle differences.

Incidence rates of fractures seem to be higher among whites than among nonwhites regardless of the geographic area involved, a possible indication that the variation is more closely related to race. Rochester, Minnesota is preponderantly populated with persons of Northern European extraction. Fracture rates are high for similar ethnic groups in Sweden, New Zealand, and South Africa. The incidence of hip fractures is very low for the Maori people in New Zealand and the Bantu in South Africa. Conversely, rates are relatively high among the caucasoid Indians in Singapore, an otherwise low incidence area. European- and American-born Jewish women in Jerusalem have higher rates of hip fracture than do women in that city of Asian or African descent or those who are native-born Israelis. Age-related fractures are generally thought to be uncommon among blacks in the United States, although epidemiologic documentation of this point is weak. The crude hospital dismissal rate for hip fractures for nonwhites, as calculated by using the aforementioned national data, is only 36 percent of that for whites. The median age for nonwhites in the United States in 1970, however, was much less (22.7 years) than that for whites (28.9 years); and the dismissal rates could not be age-adjusted. Thus, the true ratio of rates is probably somewhat greater than the figure noted. More specific studies of fracture rates by race in the United States have involved too few nonwhites to be convincing.

The pattern of incidence of fractures of the proximal femur varies by race even more dramatically than the overall rates. Among the Bantu, the incidence of hip fractures increases only minimally with advancing age, and rates for men are slightly higher than those for women.

Among Chinese and Malay residents of Singapore, rates for males are also higher than those for women; but the incidence among both sexes does rise modestly with increasing age. The pattern for Indian residents of Singapore resembles that of Western men and women. A similar pattern has been observed for Colles' fracture in Singapore. Singapore is also unusual in that 26 percent of the men and 11 percent of the women were under the age of 50 years at the time of hip fracture. Such an event is unusual in the West. In Rochester, Minnesota, for example, only 4 percent of the patients of both sexes with hip fracture were younger than 50 years old. In Jerusalem, women have a greater incidence rate than men for each of the three cultural groups mentioned before, but the difference is less notable for those of Asian and African extraction. Among the Maori in New Zealand, men and women have similar incidence rates of hip fractures.

The true reasons for these differences are unknown, although speculation is rife. Racial differences in bone density have been described, with American blacks said to have substantially greater levels of bone density than whites of the same age and sex. The Bantu, however, who have the lowest reported incidence rates of hip fractures of any population, are reported to have values for metacarpal bone density that are actually lower than those of Johannesburg whites, who display the usual Western pattern of hip fracture incidence. Dietary explanations are inconsistent as well. The incidence of fracture of the proximal femur was greater in a rural area of Yugoslavia with low calcium consumption than it was in an area with high calcium consumption, but other dietary differences were noted for the two areas. Unexpectedly, perhaps, the incidence of fractures of the distal forearm did not differ significantly between the high and low calcium regions. In general, areas that seem to be deficient in dietary calcium, protein, and vitamin D have lower fracture rates, whereas the incidence is highest in the developed countries where diets are "better." Deaths from falls are reportedly less common in areas with naturally fluoridated water than in other regions, but such mortality data are very unreliable. A protective effect of hard physical labor has been hypothesized to explain the low incidence of hip fractures among Chinese women and the Bantu of both sexes. Convincing data for such a conclusion do not exist, although exercise seems to influence bone mass. The adverse effects of immobilization and weightlessness on bone mass are well recognized.

All of these hypotheses may be misleading, however. In the first place, fractures may be a relatively insensitive index to subtle variations in the patterns of bone loss among ethnic groups. Certainly, the differential exposure to trauma associated with age, sex, occupation, social class, and so forth complicates interpretation of the data. More importantly, few studies have been based on the comprehensive evaluation of fractures in patients and appropriate control subjects from the different racial groups. The observations reported to date may have resulted from the "ecologic fallacy" whereby the characteristics of entire populations are attributed to the actual patients with hip fracture, who, in fact, may differ considerably from the overall population. Convincing explanations for the apparent racial differences await more detailed study of fracture cases and control subjects in the various geographic regions.

Diminished Bone Density

Obviously, some cases of osteoporosis and resultant fractures can be ascribed to specific underlying diseases (secondary osteoporosis), whereas no such cause can be identified in other cases (primary or idiopathic osteoporosis). This does not mean, of course, that the primary cases are without cause; as with other conditions, the proportion of cases attributed to idiopathic osteoporosis will undoubtedly decline as knowledge accumulates. In the interim, it should be possible to identify factors, such as leanness or smoking, that are associated with an enhanced risk of osteoporosis and to use these features to identify candidates for closer evaluation or prophylactic treatment. This pragmatic epidemiologic approach has proved useful for initiating control measures for other diseases, even in the absence of a thorough understanding of the underlying pathophysiology.

On the basis of the presented material, female sex, advancing age, and white race clearly seem to be associated with an increased risk of fracture, and therefore could be called risk factors. These attributes, however, are so broad that they provide relatively little help in identifying specific high-risk subgroups in the population. Numerous other conditions have been suggested as risk factors for or causes of reduced bone density, but few of these putative risk factors have been well documented from the epidemiologic standpoint. Many have never been studied with epidemiologic methods at all. This deficiency is important to note because fundamental problems exist with much of the data currently available for evaluating risk. For example, studies based on series of referral patients are unlikely to reflect accurately the true importance of various risk factors in the community because unusual conditions are generally overrepresented. Thus, although the therapeutic use of corticosteroids in severe juvenile rheumatoid arthritis can undoubtedly lead to hip fractures that are obviously abnormal, this must be a rare cause of hip fracture in the general population.

It is also difficult to decide from the information available whether particular conditions are risk factors or not. Even when all patients with hip fracture in a population are studied, half or more will be found to have a chronic disease. Because the median age of patients with hip fracture is about age 70, however, such conditions would be expected to be quite common. Without a proper control group, one cannot determine which of these conditions is more frequent than expected. Diabetes mellitus is a case in point. The very occurrence of a hip fracture may impose sufficient stress to alter glucose metabolism to the point where diabetes could be diagnosed, even if only transiently. This factor would elevate the observed frequency of diabetes among the cases. Even if a prior history of diabetes was demanded before each case was counted, adequate control data are rarely available. One study of patients with hip fracture compared the number of cases of diabetes observed with the number expected on the basis of age- and sex-specific diabetes prevalence rates in the population. The diabetes prevalence rates were from a pilot survey, however, and were later found to be too low. Thus, the calculated expected prevalence of diabetes was then also too low, and diabetes was spuriously identified as a risk factor for hip fracture. In Rochester, Minnesota, a retrospective cohort study was conducted by using all of the incidence cases of diabetes ($N = 1135$) that were diagnosed in the population, and observing both prior and subsequent fractures in comparison with an age- and sex-matched control cohort of nondiabetics from the general population. As would be anticipated, the diabetic patients had no greater incidence of fracture before diagnosis. Unexpectedly, the incidence of fractures after the diagnosis of diabetes was not elevated either. This finding was consistent for various clinical types of diabetes diagnosed at different ages and for various types of fractures, including the age-related fractures. Thus, despite animal and some human evidence of osteopenia associated with diabetes, diabetes mellitus did not seem to increase the risk of fracture in this relatively large cohort study.

Even when adequate control groups have been included, however, few studies have employed methods suitable for assessing the actual risk associated with any specific factor. Typically, the proportion of patients who have a particular characteristic is compared with the proportion of control subjects who have it. Thus, chronic alcoholism may be 5 to 10 times more frequent among patients with fractures than among control subjects. The disproportion may be even greater for appreciable use of corticosteroids. In comparison with control subjects, about twice as many patients with fractures are likely to smoke or have a history of gastrectomy, hyperthyroidism, or renal failure, and about 1.5 times as many patients may have a history of bilateral oophorectomy or long immobilization. The reported association between fractures and peptic ulcer disease seems primarily accounted for by the effect of gastrectomy, and that of rheumatoid arthritis may be due to the use of corticosteroids. As previously noted, diabetes mellitus does not appear to be an important factor. In contrast, less than four-fifths as many patients as control subjects usually have a history of postmenopausal estrogen use, and only one-third as many are obese. Even though the evaluation of such differences between patients and control subjects is an appropriate analytic technique in many clinical studies, this is not the proper method of assessing the actual risk due to any putative causal factor. As noted in the section on methodology, risk is measured by the odds ratio in case-control studies or by the relative risk in a cohort study.

The investigation of diabetes mellitus and subsequent fractures that was previously mentioned is one of the few cohort studies in this area. Several case-control studies have been undertaken, primarily to assess the protective effects of postmenopausal use of estrogen. Some of these studies have had serious methodologic flaws that raise questions about the results obtained. Nonetheless, postmenopausal use of estrogen apparently does exert a protective effect against age-related fractures. An estimated relative risk of fracture of 0.8 or less with postmenopausal use of estrogen indicates that users have only about 80 percent of the fracture risk of nonusers. The protective effect seems to increase with greater duration of postmenopausal estrogen therapy and to be greater for some subgroups of women, such as those who have had oophorectomy. In most of these studies, obesity has exerted an independent protective effect.

Other conditions have been found among patients with fractures, but the actual magnitude of the risk, if any, associated with each is unknown. In general, one would anticipate that the risk of any specific factor would be greater for men than women. This probably results from the higher background level of idiopathic osteoporosis among women. Additionally, investigators have observed that younger patients with age-related fractures are more likely to have an underlying illness and that, conversely, patients with secondary osteoporosis are likely to have fractures at a somewhat younger age. Clinical evidence is persuasive for a relationship between diminished bone density and factors such as hyperparathyroidism, hemiplegia, immobilization, hypercortisonism, use of corticosteroid, malabsorption syndrome, pelvic irradiation therapy, uremia, dialysis, anticonvulsant therapy, menopause, and male hypogonadism. Although epidemiologic evidence regarding the mechanisms through which such risk factors might influence bone density is essentially nonexistent, a wealth of knowledge has been gained through other means and detailed in Chapter 7. Other conditions, such as urolithiasis, are probably not risk factors in themselves but serve only as markers of some other abnormality of bone metabolism. Further research is necessary to document the role of a final list of conditions observed among patients with fracture, including Parkinsonism, hypertension, atherosclerosis, chronic anticoagulation therapy, pulmonary tuberculosis, chronic obstructive lung disease, chronic liver disease, and others. Many of these associations may simply be coincidental.

Propensity for Trauma

Elderly patients actually have a lower incidence of medically attended injuries each year than do young adults, but they are hospitalized more frequently and die as a result of the injury much more often. Although persons with reduced bone density may be subjected to severe trauma like anyone else, they are uniquely at risk for fractures sustained with moderate trauma of the sort that rarely results in fractures among young people. The consensus of almost all studies to date is that the degree of antecedent trauma declines as the age of the patient advances. The most common cause, by far, of fractures among elderly persons is a simple fall from a standing height or less. A third or more of all elderly individuals experience such a fall each year, and those age 65 or older account for about three-fourths of the fatal falls recorded in the United States each year.

The causes of these falls are numerous. In the individual patient, the cause is often the result of a complex interaction of several factors.

Although the true contribution of each cause of falls in the general population is uncertain, the overall pattern is reasonably clear. A half or more of the falls among elderly persons are associated with definable organic dysfunction, and the proportion increases with advancing age. The majority of victims have one or more of the many physiologic deficits associated with aging, including diminished postural control, gait changes, muscular weakness, decreased reflexes, poor vision, postural hypotension, vestibular problems, confusion, and dementia. Elderly persons are also less able to break the impact of a fall because of decreased strength and reaction time. Specific acute diseases seem to play a role in a minority of falls. Parkinsonism, stroke and hemiplegia, cardiac rhythm and conduction defects, pneumonia, arthritis, and alcoholism seem prominent. Iatrogenic problems include excessive use of sedatives leading to falls at night and overtreatment of hypertension with resulting hypotension. So-called drop attacks, postulated to result from disturbances in blood flow to brainstem postural centers, may be the cause of 10 to 20 percent of falls among elderly people.

Environmental hazards are thought to be primarily responsible for about a third of falls, although the aforementioned factors may contribute considerably. The leading hazards seem to be slippery surfaces and loose rugs, although steps, curbs, light cords, and other obstacles also lead to falls. About three-fourths of all falls occur indoors, and many are associated with merely getting in or out of a chair or bed. Falls seem to be somewhat more common during the active hours of daylight than at night, and perhaps more common in winter than in other seasons. Both environmental and seasonal variation in falls are minimized among nursing home residents and other institutionalized individuals.

These general points have been confirmed by investigations of specific age-related fractures, especially fractures of the proximal femur. Although the uncommon hip fractures among young people are likely to be associated with severe trauma, most hip fractures occur among older persons, and about 9 of 10 are associated with only moderate or minimal trauma. A few of these fractures seem to be spontaneous, and another small group are associated with specific pathologic lesions such as metastatic malignant tumors or bone cysts. Most of the fractures associated with moderate trauma, however, are due to falls. Reasons for the falls vary from study to study, depending on whether the authors emphasize the external circumstances or the patients' underlying deficits. In general, however, a third to a half are due to trip-

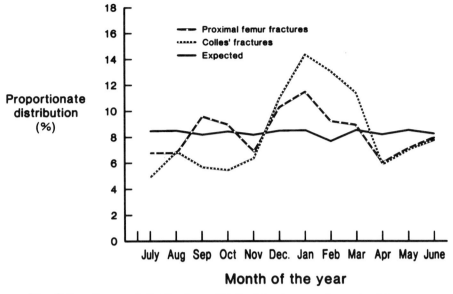

Fig. 3-5.   Seasonal distribution of Colles' fractures and proximal femur fractures among residents of Rochester, Minnesota compared with that expected if the fractures were distributed evenly from month to month.

ping or slipping, another fifth are secondary to syncope or a drop attack, a fifth to a third are due to a loss of balance, and the remainder are the result of miscellaneous factors such as collisions with others or seizures. Trips and slips may be somewhat more frequent causes of falls among the less elderly patients with hip fracture, whereas the very elderly are more likely to fall because they lose their balance or suffer a drop attack. Regardless of the exact reason for falling, about three-fourths of the fractures occur indoors; for this reason, perhaps, a seasonal pattern for hip fractures is not pronounced (Fig. 3-5). Most Colles' fractures are also due to moderate trauma, again, typically falls. These falls have not been studied in as much detail as those associated with hip fractures, but a greater proportion seem to occur outdoors. This finding is supported by the seasonal pattern of Colles' fracture (Fig. 3-5), which reveals an increased incidence in winter that is much more substantial than for hip fracture. An epidemic of such fractures associated with an ice storm has been reported.

CORRELATION OF VARIOUS AGE-RELATED FRACTURES

Perhaps the most surprising observation about the various age-related fractures is that they are not more closely correlated with each other. When the age- and sex-specific incidence rates for the major fractures are plotted on the same scale (Fig. 3-6), considerable variability is apparent. For example, the age- and sex-specific incidence rates for cervical and intertrochanteric hip fractures (which are combined in Figure 3-6) are essentially identical in Rochester, although the cervical region is composed predominantly of cortical bone (75 percent cortical and 25 percent trabecular) and the intertrochanteric region is composed of about 50 percent of each bone type. The former approximates the composition of the distal radius at the usual scanning sites, but the age- and sex-specific incidence patterns for hip and Colles' fractures are quite different. This serves to re-emphasize the point that the many interactions between bone metabolism and trauma are complex. More detailed study of such interactions may help refine pathophysiologic hypotheses to be tested in subsequent investigations of age-related fractures.

Clinical studies of patients with fractures of the hip, distal radius, proximal humerus, or vertebra have generally found some evidence of diminished bone density at the site of the fracture, especially if the fracture has occurred with only a modest degree of trauma. The epidemiologic evidence on this point is more circumstantial. For example, bone density in the upper limbs has generally been found to be less on the left side than on the right, although this difference apparently has not been found in the lower limbs. In Rochester, 57 percent of fractures of the proximal humerus and 75 percent of Colles' fractures occur on the left side, but fractures of the proximal femur are evenly divided between right and left sides. Other investigators have noted that hip fractures associated with severe trauma, and especially motor vehicle accidents, more frequently involve the left hip than the right. It has already been shown that fracture rates are greater for women, who have lower bone density levels than men, and that the rates increase with advancing age among both sexes as bone density diminishes. Furthermore, patients with one type of age-related fracture often have another type. Patients with hip fracture are about twice as likely as expected to have had a prior fracture of the proximal humerus and vice versa. Patients with hip fracture are 3 to 10 times more likely (depending on age) to

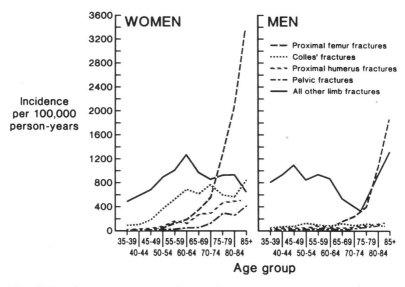

Fig. 3-6. Age- and sex-specific incidence rates for a number of age-related fractures among residents of Rochester, Minnesota, with all rates shown to the same scale.

have had a prior vertebral fracture. The likelihood of a patient with hip fracture having had a prior Colles' fracture has been estimated from population-based studies at 1.3 to 1.9 times the expected value. Similarly, patients with a Colles' fracture seem to be at about twice the normal risk for a subsequent hip fracture. Nonetheless, this correlation between different age-related fractures is much less than one would expect if all fractures were related to exactly the same underlying disorder. Even though the risk is increased significantly, the practical result is that most patients with Colles' fracture will not have a subsequent hip fracture and most patients with hip fracture will not have had a prior Colles' fracture. Thus, even though Colles' fractures become common 15 to 20 years before hip fractures do, the ability of a Colles' fracture to predict which patients will sustain subsequent hip fractures is small.

This poor correlation is partly due to varying proportions of cortical and trabecular bone at the different fracture sites and to differences in the patterns of loss of these two types of bone. These phenomena will be discussed in depth elsewhere. It may be sufficient to note here that the risk of Colles' fracture is related to the bone mineral content of the distal radius but is less closely correlated with trabecular bone density, especially among men. In contrast, patients with hip fractures seem to have both trabecular osteoporosis, as measured in the spine and the iliac crest, and cortical osteoporosis, as measured in the metacarpals. Patients with intertrochanteric hip fractures, however, are much more likely than patients with other types of hip fracture to have a recurrent fracture in the intertrochanteric region of the opposite hip, and are more likely than patients with cervical fractures to have had a previous vertebral fracture or other evidence of spinal osteoporosis. Patients with cervical fractures are more likely to have a recurrent fracture in the cervical region of the opposite hip and to have evidence of cortical osteoporosis in the metacarpals.

Patients with fractures may not be clearly distinguishable from their peers without fractures, however, because the distribution of bone density values for patients and control subjects overlaps in most studies. Age- and sex-matched control subjects cannot accurately be considered "normal" because most will have lost bone to some degree, even if they have not yet experienced a fracture. Both patients and controls typically have bone density levels less than those found among young adults who have not begun to lose bone. This finding suggests that factors other than density may affect bone fragility and that among those with equal bone fragility other forces determine who will experience a fracture. In this instance, the entire concept of normal and abnormal may be misleading. An analogy is suggested with hypertension and stroke. Those who experience a stroke cannot be completely separated from people without a stroke solely on the basis of blood pressure. Nevertheless, the risk of stroke clearly increases as blood pressure increases. Likewise, the risk of fracture apparently increases as bone density declines, though the magnitude of the risk at each level of bone density has not yet been determined.

PROSPECTS FOR PROPHYLAXIS

Although there is evidence that elderly people fall frequently, the greater problem is the prevalence in this age group of bones weakened by osteoporosis. The occurrence of falls could possibly be reduced by identifying factors that could be emphasized in educational and safety programs directed toward elderly persons and by recognizing high-risk medical practices—e.g., inappropriate use of antihypertensive drugs in elderly patients. The most promising avenue, however, is prevention of excessive bone loss. As subsequent chapters indicate, there is evidence that bone loss in postmenopausal women can be prevented or retarded by therapeutic agents such as estrogens and supplemental calcium. A recent consensus conference of the National Institutes of Aging (Bethesda, Maryland, September 13–14, 1979, p 3) concluded, "Estrogen administration represents a promising approach to prevention of the widespread problem of hip fracture." Unfortunately, use of estrogen may be associated with important side effects such as endometrial carcinoma. Moreover, compliance and cost will be problems with the long-term drug administration that is probably required. These difficulties can be minimized by identifying, as candidates for preventive drug therapy, the specific subgroups of the population at greatest risk of osteoporotic fractures. Therapeutic and/or preventive programs as detailed in Chapters 7 and 8 should then be considered.

In any lengthy list of risk factors for osteoporosis, one is immediately impressed that a great many are specific clinical diagnoses, surgical procedures, or drug regimens. Falls among the elderly have been much less studied and clinical risk factors have been less well evaluated, but the same observation—that diagnoses and therapeutic regimens represent important risk factors—seems to be true for falls. Thus, many elderly patients who ultimately sustain a fracture must have had clinically evident, or even iatrogenic, factors that could have been recognized by their physicians early on and used to select a high-risk subpopulation for further evaluation with more specific techniques, such as bone densitometry, that are too expensive for routine screening. Convincing evidence for the importance of such risk factors might spur more aggressive efforts to treat or minimize the primary condition and could justify the use of preventive drug therapy despite its attendant risks. The primary challenge in the epidemiology of age-related fractures now is determining (1) which patient characteristics are actually risk factors for fractures in the general population, (2) which factors have the greatest impact on the incidence of fractures in the community, and (3) which factors can be identified early enough before the fractures to permit timely intervention. This information should lead to efficient strategies for the control of age-related fractures.

BIBLIOGRAPHY

Alffram P-A: An epidemiologic study of cervical and trochanteric fractures of the femur in an urban population: Analysis of 1,664 cases with special reference to etiologic factors. Acta Orthop Scand [Suppl] 65:1-109, 1964

Alffram P-A, Bauer GCH: Epidemiology of fractures of the forearm: A biomechanical investigation of bone strength. J Bone Joint Surg [Am] 44-A:105–114, 1962

Gallagher JC, Melton LJ, Riggs BL, Bergstralh E: Epidemiology of fractures of the proximal femur in Rochester, Minnesota. Clin Orthop 150:163–171, 1980

Garraway WM, Stauffer RN, Kurland LT, O'Fallon WM: Limb fractures in a defined population. I. Frequency and distribution. Mayo Clin Proc 54:701–707, 1979

Melton LJ, Sampson JM, Morrey BF, Ilstrup DM: Epidemiologic features of pelvic fractures. Clin Orthop 155:43–47, 1981

Rose SH, Melton LJ, Morrey BF, Ilstrup DM, Riggs BL. Epidemiologic features of humerus fractures. Clin Orthop 1982, 168:24–30

4

Noninvasive Methods for Quantitating Appendicular Bone Mass

C. Conrad Johnston, Jr.

Among methods for assessing bone mass, photon absorptiometry and radiogrammetry are the most widely available, the least costly, and the lowest in radiation dose to the patient. Each can provide valuable clinical data when properly utilized, but the limitations of the methods should be known. When choosing a technique, it is important to define the purpose for which the particular measurement is being made. Is the goal to estimate total skeletal mass and to separate the deficient individual from the normal? Or is the purpose to measure rates of bone loss to find the individual who is losing most rapidly? Or is the purpose to determine the effect of a therapeutic intervention on rate of change? Or perhaps epidemiologic studies are being done to ascertain the effect of environmental factors on change in bone mass. The specific aims of the study being done may dictate the best method to be used.

Frequently, the clinical problem being addressed is the diagnosis of osteoporosis. Commonly, an attempt may be made to identify the individual with this disease before fracture occurs. In this circumstance, the technique selected should have the greatest accuracy in discerning the quantity of bone present. An underlying assumption is that fractures, the morbid event in osteoporosis, are the result of low bone mass at the fracture sites. It is also frequently assumed that the measurements made in the appendicular skeleton by the techniques discussed here reflect bone mass at sites where the fractures occur. Neither of these assumptions is entirely correct. Certainly low bone mass is a major factor contributing to fracture pathogenesis, but other abnormalities intrinsic or extrinsic to the skeleton must play a role as well. Disturbances in bone remodeling and other disease such as osteomalacia also predispose to fracture. Muscle weakness and neurologic disorders may lead to an increased frequency of falling, and certainly, the degree and frequency of trauma is also an important determinant of fracture; i.e., not all individuals with low bone mass have fractures, the clinical syndrome of osteoporosis, and thus no measurement of skeletal mass will always identify those who will experience fracture. The best expectation is to discern those with greatest risk of fracture.

Bone mass as measured at a peripheral site by radiogrammetry or by photon absorptiometry may not accurately reflect mass in other parts of the skeleton or in the entire skeleton. These methods primarily measure cortical bone, and in some individuals the trabecular bone of the spine may be lost rapidly; thus these deficits would not be identified in peripheral cortical bone. Conversely, when low bone mass is found at any measured site, there probably has been a general loss of bone. A normal value in the periphery does not exclude low bone mass in other loci such as the spine.

The quantity of bone present in the aging skeleton is influenced by many factors: among them, age, sex, race, and body size. Each factor contributes to variation of bone mass found in populations of all ages, and such variation increases the difficulty in separating normal from abnormal. Statistical techniques have been developed for partially removing the effects of these variables. This process is sometimes called normalization. Normalization should be used when the goal is to determine whether an individual or individuals have normal or abnormal bone mass.

Another major use of bone mass measurement is for following changes in bone mass. In this circumstance the primary aims may be to identify individuals losing bone at the greatest rates or to ascertain the effects of therapeutic intervention on bone loss or gain. In these situations, the rates of change in cortical bone will probably be small. Normal postmenopausal women lose 1 to 2 percent of cortical bone per year. Thus, the method with the greatest precision should be chosen. An assumption is that changes in the measured site reflect changes in the total skeleton or, at least, in other sites of interest. As noted, this assumption may not be correct. Trabecular bone of the spine may be more rapidly lost or gained than peripheral cortical bone. Nevertheless, the direction of change throughout the skeleton is usually the same,

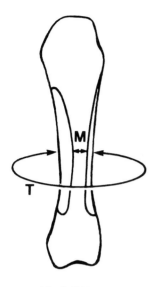

Fig. 4-1. Measurements of total width (T) and medullary width (M) of metacarpal.

even if of different magnitude. If an individual is found to be losing bone rapidly at a measured site, it is usually concluded that bone is being lost at other loci, but not always at the same rate.

RADIOGRAMMETRY

Morphometric measurements can be made on all peripheral tubular bones, but the most common site is the metacarpal, or several metacarpal bones. Radiogrammetry is simple, readily available, and normative data is abundant in the literature. It can be utilized routinely for evaluating the response to therapeutic programs. A standard posterioanterior radiograph, using nonscreen film, is made of the hand. Sequential studies require that the hand be repositioned similarly for each measurement and that the x-ray tube-film distance remain constant.

A measurement of total width and medullary width at the midshaft of the metacarpal is made (Fig. 4-1). Needle-tipped Vernier calipers are needed for the most accurate measurements. In addition, it is ideal if one observer makes the measurements and if a series of films of the same individual is measured at the same time. Most often the second metacarpal bone has been used for measurement, but if maximum precision is required for sequential studies, measurements of the second, third, and fourth metacarpal bones of both hands are needed.

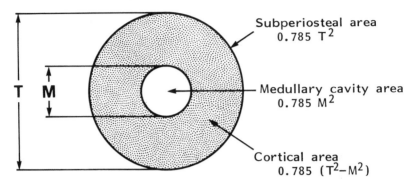

Fig. 4-2.   Calculation of subperiosteal area, medullary cavity area, and cortical area of metacarpal.

   If it is assumed that the bone is a regular cylinder, additional calculations of the area within the periosteum and of the area of the medullary canal can be made (Fig. 4-2). Ratios of cortical area to total area can be determined and the percent cortical area calculated. It is also possible to measure the length of the metacarpal bone. Some investigators have used this measurement to normalize for body size.
   When this technique is used, the width of cortical bone present is measured. No evaluation of trabecular bone is possible, and changes that occur within the Haversian envelope, the bone between periosteum and endosteum, are not measured. Thus, increased cortical porosity, which occurs in some diseases and with aging, is not detected. Quantitatively, the majority of bone that is lost from tubular bones with aging is due to endosteal resorption. Growth continues to occur on the periosteal surface throughout life. Radiogrammetry is well suited for detecting these changes.
   Radiogrammetry is only moderately accurate in reflecting the amount of bone present at the measured site. Correlations of the order of r = 0.6 to 0.7 have been reported. The cortical area correlates better with the amount of bone present than does cortical width. The precision of this technique is 5 to 10 percent on measurements of a single metacarpal bone, but 1 to 3 percent using multiple measurements of six metacarpal bones. Measurements in the metacarpals do not correlate well with measurements in other peripheral bones (r = 0.5 to 0.7), and even less well with trabecular bone of the iliac crest and with total body calcium as measured by neutron activation. Thus, radiogrammetry is not a good technique for estimating total skeletal mass or the quantity of trabecular bone in the spine or iliac crest.

Advantages of the radiogrammetric technique, especially as applied to metacarpals, are its simplicity, its wide availability at reasonable cost, its relatively good precision, and its ability to measure changes on the endosteal and periosteal surfaces. Disadvantages include limited accuracy, poor correlation with other measurements of cortical or trabecular bone and total body calcium, and failure to measure porosity, which develops in the Haversian envelope with disease and age.

PHOTON ABSORPTIOMETRY

The technique of photon absorptiometry utilizes a well collimated beam of mono-energetic radiation, usually from ^{125}I, to scan a peripheral bone. The intensity of the beam is monitored with a collimated scintillation detector. A limb is immersed in water or wrapped with a water bag or tissue-equivalent material to provide equal soft tissue cover. The amount of skeletal mineral present is proportional to change in beam intensity over the bone (Fig. 4-3). Calculations of bone mass in gm/cm can then be made if the density and mass absorption coefficients are known, or if a proper standard is utilized. An instrument can be constructed from components, but commercial units that provide a direct read-out of bone mass are also available.

Photon absorptiometry minimizes the effects of scattered radiation and beam hardening that contribute to the inaccuracy of radiographic techniques. It provides an accurate assessment of the amount of mineral (correlation coefficient r = 0.98, error of estimate, 5–6 percent). It should be noted that the total amount of mineral in the scan path is measured, and if change occurs over time, net change is detected. This technique does not measure endosteal or periosteal surfaces, as does radiogrammetry, but it does detect change on all surfaces: periosteal, endosteal, and Haversian.

Although any peripheral bone can be measured, the most widely studied sites are the radius and/or ulna. Thus, a variety of normative data are available for comparison. Scans must be performed at the same site to allow comparison between groups. In addition, since there is genetic variation in bone mass, and genetic mixes of specific populations may vary, it is essential that an adequate number of normal individuals of different ages be studied to provide a normal range.

The precision of repeated measurements is quite good: 1 to 2 percent in the research laboratory and 2 to 5 percent in the clinical setting. The principal determinant of precision is repositioning for measure-

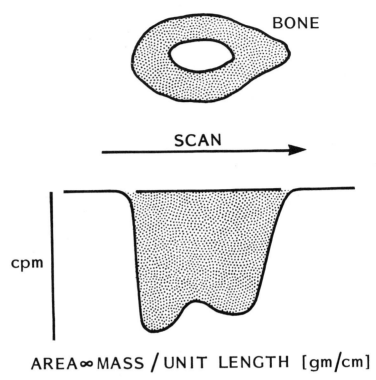

Fig. 4-3. Model of a scan of an appendicular bone using photon absorptiometry.

ment at the same site on repeated scans. Variations in marrow fat may also introduce errors, especially in trabecular bone, but this variable is primarily a problem for population studies. There is probably little change in this constituent in an individual who is followed over several years. Precision can be improved by scanning in a skeletal area where there is little change in shape or quantity of bone over several centimeters of its length. This requirement is met by the midshaft of the radius. In this location minor differences in positioning are of lesser importance. An arm-holder to firmly fix the limb in the same position, or a plaster cast of the limb, made for each individual, are useful for exact repositioning. This approach leads to improved precision. Another way to improve precision is by area scanning or making several scans close together along the bone and thereby giving an integrated bone mass over some distance.

Precision is important if the goal is to detect small changes such as the 1 to 2 percent per year loss found in postmenopausal women. In addition to repositioning the limb accurately, it is also necessary to make multiple measurements. In order to accurately construct rates of change for individuals, measurements should be made at least three times a year over a two-year span. Of course, if change in bone mass is more rapid or measurements are made more frequently, a shorter time span may be sufficient.

When the rate of change is to be calculated for an individual, the greatest precision is necessary and the bone mass measurements themselves, uncorrected for other variables such as body size, should be used. When an attempt is made to separate the abnormal patient from the normal population, however, the effect of other variables known to influence bone mass must be taken into account. Among these variables are age, sex, and body size. Several indices of skeletal size can be used to reduce variance, including the bone width measured from the scan, height, and body weight. The statistical procedure of multiple regression analysis is used to reduce variation caused by these factors. If only one index of skeletal size is to be used to reduce variances, the bone mass can be divided by the bone width.

The usual measurement site in the midradius contains almost entirely cortical bone, and a measure of trabecular bone may be of clinical interest. The most distal radius and ulna contain up to 70 percent trabecular bone, but this percent rapidly decreases when moving proximally. In addition, the radius is very irregular in shape at the distal end; thus repositioning is difficult and precision is reduced. In prospective studies, whatever advantage is gained by measuring at the distal site that contains the more active trabecular bone is probably lost in reduced precision.

Other bones, such as the calcaneus (which has a high content of trabecular bone), have been studied, but little normative data are available, and changes found may not reflect changes in the spine, which is generally the trabecular site of greatest interest.

There is good correlation between cortical bone mass measured in the radius and other cortical sites, such as the neck of the femur ($r = 0.85$). Radial bone mass and total body calcium measured by neutron activation correlate well in normals ($r = 0.85$), but less well in individuals with spinal osteoporosis.

The technique of photon absorptiometry has the advantage of good accuracy, precision, and wide availability at a moderate cost. For measurements made in the radius, there is good correlation with other cortical sites and with total body calcium. The method, as currently used, primarily reflects change in cortical bone; thus changes found by this technique are not a good index of changes in the trabecular bone of the spine. In addition, net changes in bone mass are measured, and specific changes on periosteal or endosteal envelopes cannot be detected.

CONCLUSIONS

As generally utilized, the methods described here—radiogramme-try and single energy photon absorptiometry—measure primarily cortical bone. In some sites (the most distal radius and the calcaneus), trabecular bone is measured; but changes in these areas may not always reflect what is occurring in the spine, and precision of repeated measurements is decreased because of problems of repositioning. Measurements of cortical bone in and of themselves are of clinical importance. Eighty percent of the skeleton is cortical bone, and its loss is important in the pathogenesis of fracture. Hip fractures may be primarily caused by a loss of cortical bone, and it has been suggested that even in the spine, the small amount of cortex present provides much of the strength of the vertebrae. Age-related bone loss occurs from both trabecular and cortical compartments, and the direction of change (if not the rate) is similar in each. With some forms of therapy, however, more rapid change occurs in the trabecular component; thus measurement of trabecular bone would detect change sooner. Nevertheless, it is important to monitor change in cortical bone as well, since a therapeutic agent may produce a positive effect in trabecular bone and an adverse effect in cortical bone.

Attempts have been made to separate patients with spinal osteoporosis from controls utilizing the photon absorption technique. Figure 4-4 illustrates the significant overlap in radial bone mass measurements that is found in a population of women with and without crush fractures. As noted above, no method can be expected to absolutely separate those with fracture from normals, since factors other than low bone mass play a role in fracture pathogenesis. Measures of trabecular bone in the spine probably will provide a better separation from normal of those with vertebral fracture or high risk of fracture than will peripheral bone-mass measurements, but overlap will not be

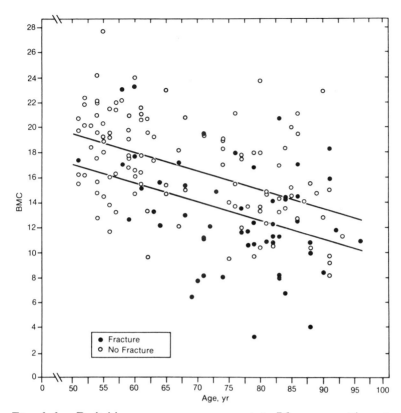

Fig. 4-4. Radial bone mass measurements in 56 women with vertebral fracture (closed circles) and 113 controls (open circles). Regression lines are significantly different. (From Smith DM, Johnston, Jr., CC, Pao-Lo Y: In vivo measurement of bone mass: Its use in demineralized states such as osteoporosis. JAMA 219:325–329, 1972, with permission.)

eliminated. A normal peripheral bone mass does not preclude low spinal mass, but a low peripheral value is probably associated with low spinal mass as well. Scans at the most distal radius reflect a larger component of trabecular bone, and bone at the distal site is lost more rapidly than in the more proximal radius. Distal radial measurement may better separate patients with spinal osteoporosis from normals than will more proximal scans. It has been shown that patients with corticosteroid induced osteoporosis have lower bone mass at the distal scan site

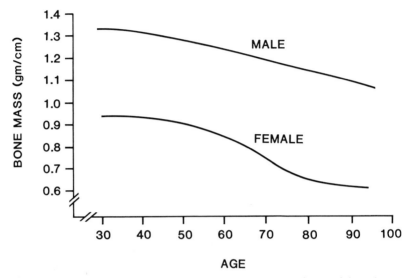

Fig. 4-5. A model of age-related bone loss in males and females.

than at the midshaft site. Because of problems of precision, however, the distal site is not best for repeated measurements.

The photon absorption technique is good for prospective studies of age-related bone loss. The patterns of bone loss in women and men is illustrated in Figure 4-5. At all ages men have more bone than women and loss is more gradual. Bone loss begins in the fourth or fifth decades in both sexes. Among women, there is an accelerated rate of loss starting around age 50 (in close association with the menopause) and there is subsequent slowing of loss. These differences in skeletal mass and rates of loss probably explain the difference in prevalence of osteoporotic fractures in the two sexes. It is hoped that generation of accurate models of age-related bone loss will allow a prediction at skeletal maturity of which segment of the population will be subsequently at greatest risk of low bone mass and increased incidence of fracture. Such predictions for individuals are not possible with the present state of our knowledge.

Both radiogrammetric and photon absorptiometric techniques have been utilized in large epidemiologic studies designed to ascertain the effects of such variables as age, race, sex, dietary calcium intake, and exercise on bone mass. The influence of age and sex has been discussed above. It has been shown also that there is a strong genetic influence on the amount of bone attained at maturity. The influences of exercise and calcium intake are somewhat more controversial and require further study. Both techniques have been utilized to test the effect of therapeutic intervention on subsequent rates of bone loss. For example, it has been shown that the administration of estrogen to oophorectomized or postmenopausal women slows or stops cortical bone loss for some years.

Photon absorptiometry, especially as used in the radius, is perhaps a better technique for prospective studies because of its accuracy and the better correlation of the radial measurements with other sites of cortical bone and with total body calcium. This is especially true where limited numbers of patients can be studied. On the other hand, radiogrammetry, because of its wide availability, can be used in large epidemiologic studies. The two techniques are complementary, since photon absorptiometry measures net change at the site scanned including all envelopes, and radiogrammetry allows a determination of whether the endosteal or periosteal envelope was affected. For example, using the photon absorption technique in young insulin-dependent diabetics, a net deficiency of bone is found when compared to controls. And, it can be determined with radiogrammetry that this deficiency is due, in part, to a failure to attain sufficient bone on the endosteal surface during adolescent growth.

Both radiogrammetry and photon absorptiometry are widely available, reasonably inexpensive techniques, with little radiation exposure to the patient. Each measures primarily cortical bone in a peripheral site, but loss of cortical bone is an important contributing factor to osteoporotic fractures. Photon absorptiometric measurements in the radius, because of the greater accuracy and correlation with other sites of cortical bone and with total body calcium, are best for separating the abnormal patient from the normal and for prospective studies of change in bone mass when relatively small numbers of subjects are available for study. Radiogrammetry is useful in large-scale epidemiologic and therapeutic studies. The two techniques are complementary, since with photon absorptiometry, net change on all surfaces is detected, while with radiogrammetry, changes on the endosteal and periosteal surfaces can be measured. Since trabecular bone of the spine may be lost (or gained under therapeutic influences) at different rates from peripheral cortical bone, neither technique will always reflect the current status of spinal bone mass when the measurement is made.

BIBLIOGRAPHY

Cameron JR, Mazess RB, Sorenson JA: Precision and accuracy of bone mineral determination by direct photon absorptiometry. Invest Radiol 3:11–20, 1968

Christiansen C, Rödbro P, Jensen H: Bone mineral content in the forearm measured by photon absorptiometry—principles and reliability. Scand J Clin Lab Invest 35:323–330, 1975

Dequeker J: Bone and aging. Ann Rheum Dis 34:100–115, 1975

Garn SM: The Earlier Gain and the Later Loss of Cortical Bone in Nutritional Perspective. Springfield, IL, C. C. Thomas, 1970, pp 146

Hodgkinson A, Knowles CF: Laboratory methods, in Nordin BEC (ed): Calcium Phosphate and Magnesium Metabolism. New York, Churchill Livingstone, 1976, pp 525–578

Manzke, E, Chesnut III CH, Wergedal JE, Baylink, DJ, Nelp WB: Relationship between local and total bone mass in osteoporosis. Metabolism 24:605–615, 1975

Mazess RB: Noninvasive measurement of bone, in Uriel S, Barzel (ed): Osteoporosis II, New York, Grune & Stratton, 1979, pp 5–26

Nordin BEC, Horsman A, Aaron J: Diagnostic procedures, in Nordin BEC (ed): Calcium Phosphate and Magnesium Metabolism. New York, Churchill Livingstone, 1976, pp 469–524

Schlenker RA, VonSeggen WW: The distribution of cortical and trabecular bone mass along the lengths of the radius and ulna and the implications for *in vivo* bone mass measurements. Calcif Tissue Res 20:41–52, 1976

Smith DM, Norton JA, Jr, Khairi MRA, Johnston CC, Jr: The measurement of rates of mineral loss with aging. J Lab Clin Med 87:882–892, 1976

Smith DM, Khairi MRA, Norton JA, Jr, Johnston CC, Jr.: Age and activity effects on rate of bone mineral loss. J Clin Invest 56:716–721, 1976

Smith DM, Khairi MRA, Johnston CC, Jr: The loss of bone mineral with aging and its relationship to risk of fracture. J Clin Invest 56:311–318, 1975

5

Noninvasive Methods for Quantitating Trabecular Bone

Richard B. Mazess

CLINICAL MEASUREMENT

Until recently noninvasive methods permitted measurement only of compact bone in the appendicular skeleton. Those techniques have been described in depth in Chapter 2 and 4. These methods have been useful for doing clinical research on metabolic bone disease, but they often lack the sensitivity that is necessary for clinical management (diagnosis and monitoring), a sensitivity that only can be attained by measurement of trabecular bone, particularly that of the axial skeleton. Diagnostic sensitivity is dependent on accurate measurement of fracture-sensitive areas such as the spine and femoral neck, both of which have a high percentage of purely trabecular bone. It also is highly dependent on the ability to normalize such measurement values so that discrimination of abnormal cases can be readily made. On the other hand, it is not necessary to have absolute accuracy of measurement at sites of fracture risk for sequential monitoring purposes, rather it is desirable to have precise (< 2 to 5% error *in vivo*) measurements at several anatomic locations (to average out effects of locational variability). If such measurement can be done in areas of fracture risk, this is obviously an added advantage.

85

LOCATIONAL SPECIFICITY

In normal young adults there is a very high intercorrelation (r > 0.9) among areas of compact bone, a moderate degree of intercorrelation (r ~ 0.7 to 0.8) among areas of trabecular bone, and a slightly lower degree of association (r ~ 0.6 to 0.7) between areas of compact and trabecular bone. Some areas of trabecular bone, such as the os calcis, are poorly correlated with other such areas (r < 0.4). Some areas of compact bone, particularly the metacarpals, are poorly correlated with the spine and areas of trabecular bone. Other areas of compact bone, the radius, for example—provide reasonable prediction of femoral neck mass. With aging and with bone disease, the degree of association among these areas decreases, and the errors of prediction increase. In part this is a result of preferential loss in trabecular bone of the axial skeleton. In normal subjects it is possible to predict spinal status with an error of 15 percent from measurements at other locations, but in bone disease the error increases to at least 30 percent (Fig. 5-1).

The errors in prediction of trabecular bone are large even for measurements of total skeletal mass, since 80 percent of the total skeleton is compact bone. The correlation between total body calcium (by neutron activation) and trabecular bone volume (TBV) of iliac crest biopsy is only about 0.2, and the error in predicting lumbar bone mineral from total body bone mineral (by ^{153}Gd absorptiometry) is 18 percent. Consequently, accurate assessment of the status of the spine or femoral neck in bone disease requires direct measurement of those areas. A predictive error of 15 to 25 percent is not adequate for clinical purposes, since this is on the order of one standard deviation in the measured parameters. Locational specificity is particularly important for diagnostic assessments, but of less import for serial monitoring.

RESPONSIVITY OF TRABECULAR BONE

There is now clear evidence that trabecular bone not only has higher surface area and turnover than compact bone but that the net changes of bone mass that occur with disease and its therapy have an earlier onset and greater magnitude there. The accentuated bone loss that is characteristic of osteoporosis, for example, occurs earlier and is greater in the trabecular bone of the lumbar spine than in compact long

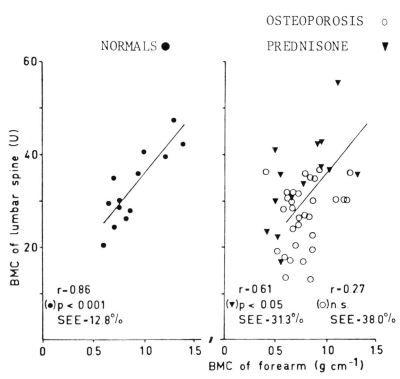

Fig. 5-1. Radius bone mineral content versus lumbar bone mineral content (by dual-photon absorptiometry) in normal subjects (left) and patients (right). The predictive error increases in the latter group (from Krølner B, Pors Nielsen S, Lund B, Lund BJ, Sorensen OH, Uhrenholdt A: Measurement of bone mineral content (BMC) of the lumbar spine, II. Correlation between forearm BMC and lumbar spine BMC. Scand J Clin Lab Invest 40:665–670, 1980).

bones. Responses to therapeutic modalities for osteoporosis seem in some cases (e.g., vitamin-D metabolites, PTH-fragment) to be wholly limited to trabecular bone, while in other cases (fluoride) the dominant effect is on trabecular bone. Similarly, vitamin-D treatment for renal osteodystrophy and for osteomalacia seems to have its most marked effect on trabecular bone. The reason for this greater responsiveness of trabecular bone and of vertebral trabecular bone in particular is not clear. The most common supposition is that the much greater specific surface area of trabecular bone provides a greater locus for cellular activity than compact bone. Moreover the blood supply to trabecular bone is many times that to compact bone. An additional physiological explanation seems to be that the major bone cells are derived from progenitor cells in the hematopoietic marrow. Rapidity of response would depend therefore on the local proliferation of stem cells. In this regard there is abundant evidence on hematopoietic response of bone marrow; vertebral marrow is many times more responsive than marrow from other trabecular areas (perhaps because its content of hematopoietic cells is twice as high as in other trabecular areas). Factors that modulate hematopoiesis in marrow could conceivably influence the responsiveness of trabecular bone. In aging, for example, there is a decline of the hematopoietic marrow and replacement with fatty marrow. In the vertebrae about 75 percent of the marrow is hematopoietic in young adulthood. With aging this fraction declines to 50 percent, and in osteoporosis only 25 percent of the marrow is hematopoietic. These age changes in marrow fat are several times the magnitude of the bone changes. Similar age changes of marrow occur in other areas of trabecular bone (distal radius, femoral neck), but the extent of the age change is less severe since these areas have much less hematopoietic marrow (50 percent) to begin with.

AGE CHANGES

The known aging decrease of trabecular bone is not greater in magnitude than that of compact bone, but it may have an earlier onset. Nearly all anatomic studies of bone density in large series, as well as the more limited studies of trabecular bone volume from iliac crest biopsy, have shown that aging decreases begin well before middle age in both sexes. In fact males and females have a very similar concentration of bone (per unit volume) in young adulthood, and both sexes show a similar aging decline of about 1 percent annually thereafter (Fig. 5-2). The aging decline of density is accompanied by a decline of strength (Fig. 5-3). The menopause seems to superimpose a brief but high loss in women (5 to 10 percent spread over several years) that is not really evident in cross-sectional data (on density or strength) but which has been observed in longitudinal studies using noninvasive methods. These decreases of trabecular bone in both sexes do not necessarily

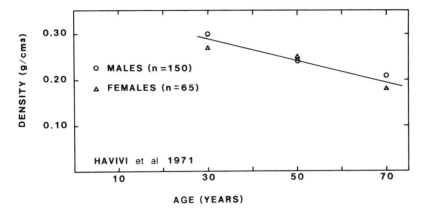

Fig. 5-2. The aging decline of trabecular bone density (200 vertebral specimens) begins in early adulthood in both sexes at a rate of about 1 percent annually (from Havivi E, Reshef A, Schwartz A, Guggenheim K, Bernstein DS, Hegsted DM, Stare FJ: Comparison of metacarpal bone loss with physical and chemical characteristics of vertebrae and ribs. Israel J Med Sci 7:1055–1062, 1971).

increase the bone specific surface and in fact the reverse may be true, since (1) the smaller and more active trabeculae are resorbed, and (2) there is a compensatory increase in the thickness of the remaining trabeculae that decreases their surface area–weight ratio. Perhaps as a consequence the bone specific uptake of radionuclides declines in trabecular bone with age, even though there is only a minor decline in blood flow. In compact bone, where both endosteal and intracortical resorption increase, the specific bone surface is increased.

The above changes of bone and marrow with aging influence the utilization of noninvasive methods to assess skeletal status. Methods that use Compton-scattering or the transmission of radiation through bone (radiographic photodensitometry, photon absorptiometry, and in particular, computed tomography) are adversely influenced by the variability of marrow composition. Radionuclide uptake methods for evaluating total skeletal dynamics are also influenced by age changes. In younger individuals a greater proportion of the uptake is accounted for by trabecular bone than is the case in either old age or osteopenic bone diseases.

Mechanical prop.

N/mm^2

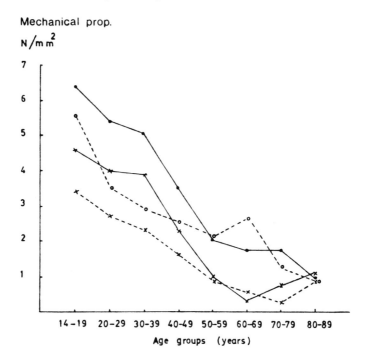

Fig. 5-3.　The decline of strength with age in males (o) and females (x) for trabecular bone from the vertebra (solid line) and tibia (dashed line) (from Lindahl O: Mechanical properties of dried defatted spongy bone. Acta Orthop Scand 47:11–19, 1976).

FRACTURES

Fracture is related to decreased bone strength, which in turn is a consequence of decreased total (not just trabecular) bone mass in these areas. Strength and resistance to fracture is directly dependent on the total mass, rather than the trabecular density. This may seem heretical, since numerous studies on trabecular bone, as well as on compact bone, have demonstrated conclusively the relationship between density and strength in anatomic samples of the same size (Fig. 5-4). The latter qualification, however, is critical, for *in vivo* bones are not of identical size. Studies on integral bone samples (femoral neck, vertebrae, distal radius) rather than small sections have shown that total mass (size times

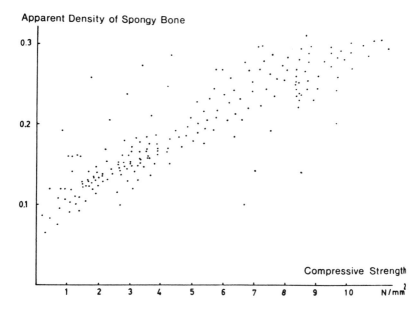

Fig. 5-4. The relationship between compressive strength and apparent density of trabecular bone (from Lindahl O: Mechanical properties of dried defatted spongy bone. Acta Orthop Scand 47:11–19, 1976).

density) is more critical for strength than either size or density alone. About 60 percent of fractured lumbar vertebrae are entirely normal in density but many may be small in size, giving them a reduced mass. In the spine vertebral strength decreases commensurate with bone mass (Fig. 5-5) as one proceeds up from the fifth lumbar vertebra, even though the apparent density of the vertebrae is relatively constant. Fractures are more common in the smaller vertebrae, however, because the degree of weight-bearing stress to which they are subject is the same as in larger vertebrae.

Much of the stress in trabecular bone seems associated with the weight-bearing function, and within the femoral neck and spine this stress appears particularly concentrated in certain regions. The vertical trabeculae in the spine and the major bundles of trabeculae in the femoral neck appear particularly important for resisting stress. Fracture may occur because (1) with bone loss the bone mass is no longer sufficient to resist ordinary stress, (2) there is too much stress as in trauma, or (3) a combination of trauma and bone loss. For example, the incidence of

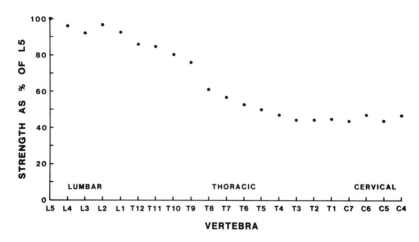

Fig. 5-5.   The variation of bone strength along the spine as a percent of the value in the fifth lumbar vertebra (adapted from Kazarian L, Graves G: Compressive strength characteristics of the human vertebral centrum Spine 2:1–14, 1977).

fractures increases by 40 percent in young adults on snowy days but by a factor of 3 (hips) to 7 (distal radius) in the elderly. Clearly there is an interaction between bone loss and trauma in producing fracture. More-over, elderly people with fractures have been shown to have experienced a higher frequency of falls as well as having lower bone mass than controls. Nevertheless, the common finding of vertebral fractures in the lower spine after menopause reflects the fact that not only is this an area of stress but also that the lumbar spine shows preferential and rapid loss of bone. Fractures occur most frequently in the upper lumbar and lower thoracic spine.

Microfractures, which appear to be harbingers of eventual verte-bral collapse, occur preferentially on the vertical trabeculae and to only a very slight extent on horizontal trabeculae (Fig. 5-6). The greatest concentration of microfractures is near the endplates of vertebrae, and in particular on L2 through L4. There is a dramatic rise in the frequen-cy of vertebral microfractures with aging (Fig. 5-7).

In general it has been found that subjects with fractures of the femoral neck have significantly reduced measurements of compact bone mass on the appendicular skeleton compared to age-matched con-trols. It is therefore surprising to note that there is little difference in trabecular bone density between the fracture group and controls (Fig.

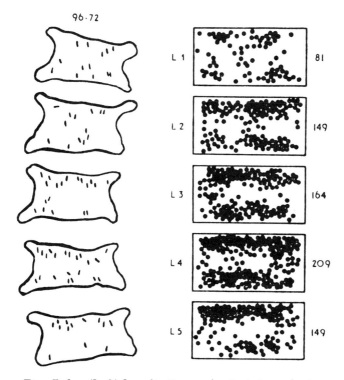

Fig. 5-6. (Left) Localization and orientation of microfractures of the lumbar spine in an 89-year-old woman. (Right) The distribution of microfractures in the lumbar vertebrae of 22 subjects. Most occur on vertical trabeculae in the superior and inferior parts of the centrum (from Vernon-Roberts B, Pirie CJ: Healing trabecular microfractures in the bodies of lumbar vertebrae. Ann Rheum Dis 32:406–412, 1973).

5-8), even when density is measured directly at the femoral neck using noninvasive methods. This would suggest that measurements of trabecular bone at this site would be of little value. One major caveat must be noted, however, for prognostic value cannot be reliably assessed from retrospective discrimination of abnormality. Besides, assessment of density does differ from measurement of mass, and it is obvious from studies *in vitro* that the total mass across the cross-section of the femoral neck is the major determinant (80 percent of variance) of strength and

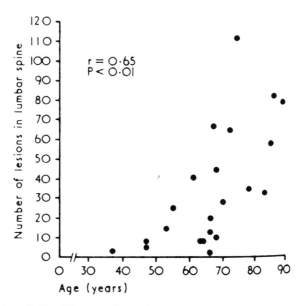

Fig. 5-7. The number of microfractures in the lumbar vertebra (22 subjects) versus age (from Vernon-Roberts B, Pirie CJ: Healing trabecular microfractures in the bodies of lumbar vertebrae. Ann Rheum Dis 32:406–412, 1973).

density is not. Hence, for diagnostic and prognostic applications, total mass is important, while for sequential measurements, "density" may be more useful in order to minimize precision errors.

Over the past decade a variety of methods have been used to examine areas of fracture-risk and to isolate the changes of trabecular bone, but only in the past several years have noninvasive methods become available that allow low-error quantitation. These methods are now used chiefly in research laboratories, but their diffusion into the clinical armatorium is expected over the next decade, and it will revolutionize diagnosis and treatment of metabolic bone diseases.

RADIOSCOPY

The oldest approach to measurement of trabecular bone changes utilized measurement or grading of the physical structures evident on radiographs. The first attempts to grade spinal radiographs systemati-

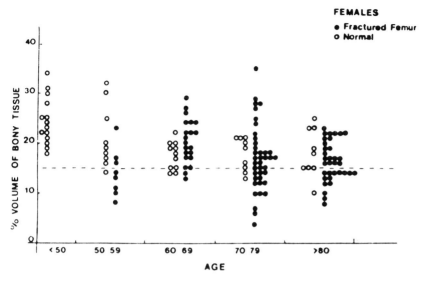

Fig. 5-8.   The trabecular bone volume in females with femoral fractures (•) compared to age-matched controls (o). The dotted line at 15 percent is the lower limit of normality in the elderly (from Aaron JE, Gallagher JC, Anderson J, Stasiak L, Longton EB, Nordin BEC Nicholson M: Frequency of osteomalacia and osteoporosis in fractures of the proximal femur. Lancet 50:229–233, 1974).

cally were made several decades ago, and various scoring procedures have been used to grade films based on the fact that optical lucency (or density) of the vertebral image is somewhat proportional to vertebral mass. This approach was hampered by the fact that optical density of the vertebral image also is dependent on exposure conditions (kilovoltage and current), scattered radiation, and film development. Approaches using step wedges, or standard vertebral specimens, exposed on the same film were a step in the right direction, but the errors remained high. The usual four or five step grading scale typically involves precision errors of two grades. A simpler approach based on measurement of vertebral height versus width, the so-called "biconcavity index," or an approach based on vertebral height compared to the height of adjacent vertebrae, also has been shown to be error-prone and insensitive. The biconcavity index is in fact poorly correlated with actual vertebral density and is not correlated with the occurrence of compression fracture.

Table 5-1
The relationship of radius bone mineral content (adjusted for width) and the Singh index of the femoral neck to (1) existing vertebral fractures, (2) other existing fractures, and (3) subsequent fractures over a three-year period. Subjects with a low radius BMC (under 0.6g/cm) had about three times the risk of subsequent fractures, while subjects with a low Singh index (grades 2 and 3) had no greater risk.

		Vertebral Fractures	Other Fractures	Subsequent Fractures
Singh Index	6	5	11	22
	5	38	13	23
	4	38	33	25
	3	85	38	54
	2	67	67	0
Adjusted BMC	>0.8	15	0	10
	0.70–0.79	39	28	33
	0.60–0.69	31	16	12
	0.50–0.59	44	19	44
	<0.5	65	40	50

Adapted from Khairi RA, Cronin JH, Robb JA, Smith DM, Johnston CC: Femoral trabecular-pattern index and bone mineral cotnent measurement by photon absorption in senile osteoporosis. J Bone Joint Surg 58:221–226, 1976.

A second approach utilized the grading of the striations visible in the proximal humerus or in the femoral neck (the Singh index). These striations correspond to the major trabecular bundles in those areas that undergo a relatively regular pattern of changes in the course of bone loss. Unfortunately the subjective grading is dependent not only on observer training but on orientation of the leg as well as film exposure and development. Consequently there is a fairly large precision error; for the seven-grade Singh index the error is typically two grades, which in fact is the difference between severely osteoporotic patients and age-matched controls. This gives the method a poor accuracy; the index is not correlated with bone mass or density in the femoral neck or at other locations. Moreover, it has been demonstrated conclusively in prospective studies that the Singh index is not of any prognostic value (Table 5-1).

These radioscopic approaches have been useful in examining grouped data for research purposes but have little applicability by themselves for routine clinical practice.

RADIOGRAPHIC PHOTODENSITOMETRY

Almost from the advent of radiography there have been efforts to extract information on bone from its radiographic image. The optical density of that image depends in part on the bone mass but, as noted in the previous section, extraneous physical factors can greatly affect the image. These factors include variations in x-ray kilovoltage and exposure, and variations in film development. These factors can be partially controlled by using simultaneous exposure of a step wedge that has absorption characteristics similar to bone. Additional factors include (1) nonuniformity of the beam over the exposed field; (2) scattered radiation, particularly in thicker body parts; and (3) preferential attenuation of the softer energies from the polychromatic x-ray beam as it passes through the body ("beam-hardening"). The last two factors have limited photodensitometry to areas of lesser soft-tissue cover (< 5cm), in particular the hand and forearm. Even in these areas, where incidentally there is very little trabecular bone, the precision of measurement has been only fair ($\sim$ 5 percent error) and the accuracy poor (5 to 15 percent error). Recent results, however, suggest that enhanced precision (3 to 4 percent) can be obtained *in vivo* by measuring large areas of the phalanges or metacarpals, thereby reducing problems of repositioning. There has been little success, however, in measuring areas containing more trabecular bone. About 20 years ago researchers at Penn State (and later at Texas Women's University) attempted to use photodensitometry to measure the trabecular bone of the os calcis, the femoral neck, and the lumbar vertebrae. The precision and accuracy were not comparable to that achieved on the hands, since with increased tissue cover, the results were degraded. Moreover, erratic results were obtained in various studies on humans, both in the evaluation of astronauts and in studies of osteoporosis.

It is possible that important trabecular areas could be measured

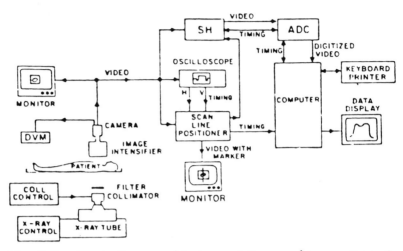

Fig. 5-9. Block diagram of instrumentation used in roentgen videoabsorptiometry for bone measurement. Scattered radiation is reduced by using scanning slits in front of the beam, and beam hardening is reduced by heavy filtration (adapted from Dobbins JT III, Mazess RB, Cameron JR: Scanning-slit x-ray videoabsorptiometry for measurement of bone mineral content. Med Phys 8:563, 1981).

despite the large amount of soft-tissue that covers them. First, it is possible to minimize the scattered radiation by using a set of scanning slits in front of the x-ray beam; these slits permit sequential exposure of small segments (a few millimeters at a time) of the total field. Second, the beam hardening can be reduced by using heavy beam filtration at high peak kilovoltage (> 100 kVp) or by using essentially monoenergetic secondary radiation from a target. These improvements have been incorporated into a roentgen videoabsorptiometry system at the University of Wisconsin (Fig. 5-9). This system uses the video signal from an image intensifier to produce a quantitative image of bone areas, thereby eliminating problems of film development. High precision and accuracy (< 2 percent) have been obtained even with heavy (20 cm) tissue cover. Such systems will become practical in radiology departments in the coming decade as a modification on the new systems for digital fluoroscopy currently being installed.

SINGLE-PHOTON ABSORPTIOMETRY

Direct photon absorptiometry was developed about 20 years ago as a transmission technique for measuring compact bone of the appendicular skeleton. A highly collimated beam (< 5mm diameter) of monoenergetic radiation from a radionuclide source (commonly ^{125}I at 27 keV or [241]Am at 60 keV) is passed across a limb, and the transmitted radiation is monitored using a collimated scintillation detector. The limb is encased in a tissue equivalent bolus (water bath, water bag, or "Super-stuff"); there must be a constant layer of tissue for the observed changes of beam intensity to be directly proportional to the bone mineral content (BMC) in the beam path. The narrow beam eliminates problems of scattered radiation while use of monoenergetic radiation minimizes the effects of selective filtration of the beam as it passes through a limb (so-called "hardening").

As discussed in the previous chapter, various attempts to apply this methodology, which is successful on compact bone, to trabecular areas have not been fruitful. First, areas such as the femoral neck and the spine cannot be readily encased in a tissue-equivalent material. Other areas, such as the distal radius, while containing far more trabecular bone than the shaft, still have a significant shell of compact bone that amounts to over 50 percent of the total mass present in a scan path. Any clinical advantages accruing from measurement at the distal radius have been offset by increased precision errors at that site. Second, trabecular areas that might be more readily measured, such as the os calcis or mandible, are less suitable for a number of technical and biological reasons. Both of the latter bones are irregular in shape, and this requires use of rectilinear scanners for accurate determination of location. Moreover, there are problems of nonuniform soft-tissue composition at these locations, as well as only modest degrees of intercorrelation (r < 0.5) with other sites of trabecular bone. Third, changes of marrow composition in trabecular areas can lead to significant problems in assessing BMC, especially with [241]Am. At the lower energy of ^{125}I, the problem is much less severe though still extant.

The os calcis measurement with rectilinear ^{125}I scanning appears a feasible means of assessing longitudinal changes of trabecular bone, though it is probably much less useful for diagnostic applications. Existing linear scanners could conceivably be modified for monitoring of the os calcis. Such monitoring has been done successfully in astronauts with better than 2 percent long-term precision; decreases of several per-

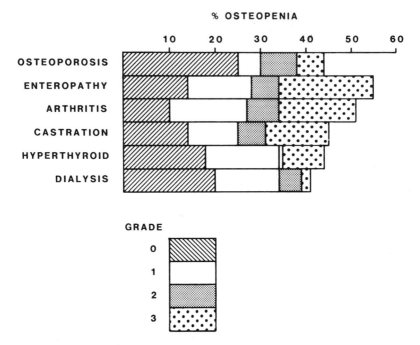

Fig. 5-10. The degree of osteopenia in the os calcis (assessed by deviancy of ^{125}I-absorptiometry values from those in normal controls). Values are shown for different conditions affecting bone and for four grades of vertebral rarefaction (0 least, 3 most). Severe vertebral osteopenia (grades 2 and 3) is reflected by a 25 percent reduction of os calcis density (adapted from Banzer DH, Schneider U, Risch WD, Botsch H: Roentgen signs of vertebral demineralization and mineral content of peripheral cancellous bone. Am J Roentgenol 126:1306–1308, 1976).

cent were demonstrated during immobilization and following space flight. Researchers at the University of Berlin have used such measurements in examining bone diseases, but the value in monitoring has yet to be demonstrated clearly; the preliminary results of a decade ago showed fairly large bone decreases after oophorectomy and increases after parathyroidectomy. The os calcis bone mineral is low in most disease with osseous involvement, and the extent of demineralization correlates with the degree of spinal osteopenia seen in radiographs (Fig. 5-10).

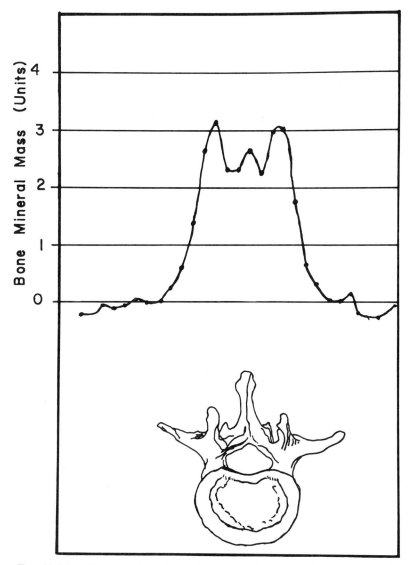

Fig. 5-11. Dual-photon absorptiometry allows the mineral mass to be calculated in scans across the vertebrae; this includes the spinous processes (50 percent of the mass). About 65 percent of the total mass is trabecular and 35 percent "compact."

DUAL-PHOTON ABSORPTIOMETRY

Some of the limitations of single-photon absorptiometry are over-come by making measurements at two distinct energies (Fig. 5-11). This eliminates the need to have a constant thickness of soft tissue around the bone and enables measurement at any body location. In addition the influence of fat variations in the marrow on the measured bone mineral is reduced.

The initial application of the dual-photon approach was for limb measurements. The sources used were a combination of ^{125}I and ^{241}Am in the U.S. and Sweden, and ^{241}Am and ^{137}Cs in England. For given counting statistics (or dose) the dual-photon approach is several times less precise than single-photon absorptiometry, so these pioneering efforts were not particularly useful. The studies did lead to later development of dual-photon approaches using ^{153}Gd (44 and 100 keV) for measurement of the spine and the femoral neck (Fig. 5-12). This source has nearly the ideal photon energies for measurements of bone through thicker soft-tissue layers. It also has a relatively long half-life (242 days), so the usual 1 Ci source can be used for scanning over an entire year. Presently ^{153}Gd scans are being done in about a dozen laboratories around the world. Most centers are doing rectilinear transmission scans of the lumbar vertebrae (Fig. 5-13). Such scans require about 30 minutes and give a radiation dose of about 5 to 15 mrem. Some centers have instituted scans of the femoral neck as well. The long-term precision *in vivo* of ^{153}Gd scans is about 2 to 3 percent at both locations. With this level of precision, direct monitoring of fracture sites can be done. The accuracy of measurement has been assessed on vertebrae in several laboratories with predictive errors ranging from 2 to 5 percent. The dual-photon method provides a measure of both compact and trabecular bone at these sites and is not a measure of purely trabecular bone. This may limit sensitivity of the method in examining changes over time. On the other hand, fracturing in both vertebrae and femora is a result of compact bone diminution as well as loss of trabecular bone, which may explain the high diagnostic sensitivity of this method.

There already has been an interesting assemblage of clinical results from dual-photon absorptiometry despite its recent inception. First, it has been shown that bone mineral of the lumbar spine provides a good discrimination between subjects with fractures and controls. Patients with compression fractures average about two standard deviations be-

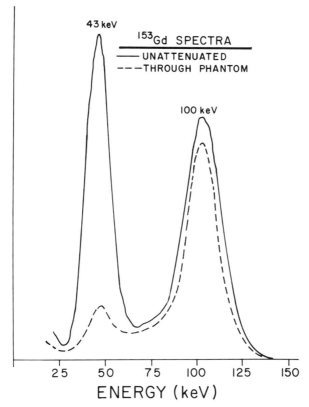

Fig. 5-12. The major source used for dual-photon absorptiometry is [153]Gd with peaks at 43 and 100 keV; in bone the lower energy peak is attenuated much more than the upper (see dashed line).

low control values, but only one standard deviation below normal in radius shaft bone-mineral content. This suggests that such patients constitute a definite subpopulation with early and/or rapid spinal bone loss. Second, subjects with femoral neck fractures have femoral neck bone mineral and radius bone mineral well below values for young adults, but their values are not greatly below those for age-matched controls. This suggests that hip-fracture patients are not a distinct subpopulation with preferential femoral neck osteopenia but rather are simply a subset of the normal aging population. Third, it has been

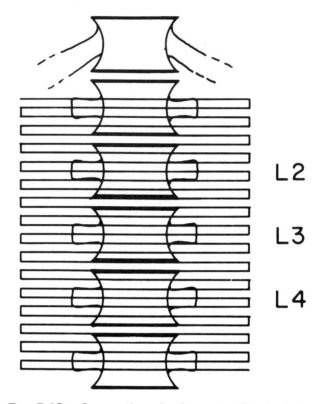

Fig. 5-13. Scan path on lumbar spine. For dual-photon absorptiometry it is usual to make a rectilinear raster scan covering at least L2 to L4 (usually with 30 to 50 scan lines). Similar scans have been made on the femoral neck.

demonstrated that sequential changes occur much more rapidly in the lumbar spine than in the compact bone of the appendicular skeleton. For example, immobilization results in a vertebral loss of 5 percent per month, compared to an expected total body calcium loss that is ten times lower. The response to various therapies (vitamin D in renal osteodystrophy and fluoride in osteoporosis) is far more rapid and marked in the lumbar spine than in the appendicular skeleton. These results indicate the value of low-error measurement at critical locations.

LOCAL NEUTRON ACTIVATION

At the beginning of the 1970s, a number of large research facilities developed methods for measuring total body calcium by neutron irradiation. The rare stable ^{48}Ca isotope, present in uniform concentration in the common ^{40}Ca, is converted to radioactive ^{49}Ca and the latter is measured in whole body counters. Calcium is a constant fraction (0.38) of bone mineral, so the ^{49}Ca can be interpreted directly as an indicator of skeletal mass in the absence of ectopic calcification (which is not the case in the elderly and in bone disease). This costly procedure has been possible in only several major centers with irradiation facilities and whole body counters. Local irradiation of the hands, forearms, and/or spine has been done in several other centers. The typical precision of these local measurements has been about 3 to 5 percent, and it is likely that the accuracy has at least a 5 percent error. The particular problems encountered are (1) high radiation dose (> 3 rem), (2) uniformity of neutron flux, and (3) uniformity in counting geometry. These problems have limited development of local activation in trabecular areas. Several laboratories have developed systems using radionuclide neutron sources (^{252}Cf or Pu-Be) to measure calcium in the spine (Fig. 5-14), while others have depended on small cyclotrons or neutron generators for neutron sources. The well-established method of trunk activation used at the University of Toronto (with Pu-Be sources) measures not only the spine but all the bone of the trunk (in an area roughly 60 x 30 cm). The dose is fairly low for activation analysis (500 mrem). This trunk measurement encompasses about 30 percent of the total skeletal calcium and hence is not specific to trabecular bone. As such it is susceptible to one major error that plagues total-body activation methods—the occurrence of ectopic calcification. Such extaosseous deposition, which is known to occur with aging and bone disease, changes the percent of calcium outside of the skeleton from perhaps 1 percent in youth to as much as 5 to 10 percent. Since much of the latter deposition occurs in the trunk area, the advantages of a trunk measurement (high percentage of trabecular bone) are offset by potential errors. Measurements limited to the spine itself (using ^{252}Cf) overcome this problem to some extent. Spinal calcium measurements do involve fairly high doses (3 rem or more), however, which prohibits their use on normal subjects, as well as inhibiting repeat measurements on patients. This dose is particularly high considering that it may involve about 50 percent of

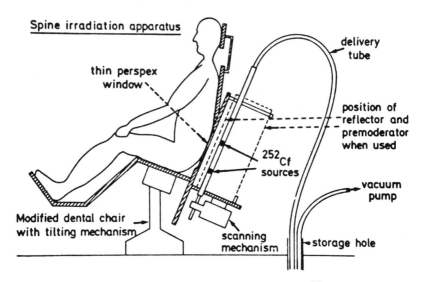

Fig. 5-14. Spinal irradiation has been done using ^{252}Cf sources with the apparatus shown (from Smith MA, Tothill P, Strong JA, Chew ISH, McIntosh LG, MacPherson JN, Simpson JD, Winney RJ: Neutron activation analysis *in vivo* of partial body calcium using Californium-252, in Mazess RB (ed): Proceedings of the Fourth International Conference on Bone Measurement. NIH Publ. No. 80-1938, 367–378, 1980).

the active marrow in the body. A lower dose is possible by using low-energy neutrons (25 keV); the technique for doing such measurements is under development at McMaster University in Canada.

COMPUTED TOMOGRAPHY

Computed axial tomography (CT) is now widely used in radiology departments for clinical imaging. There also have been efforts to make this approach quantitative in order to measure bone in both appendicular and axial skeleton. All commercial CT machines use x-ray tubes as a source of radiation, but special bone scanners have been built that use radionuclide sources (^{125}I). The basic principles of measurement, however, are similar in both x-ray and radionuclide units.

CT measurements involve making attenuation determinations at many positions in a fixed arc about an object of interest. These attenuation measurements can be done using fixed or moving sources and fixed or moving detectors (scintillation detectors or proportional counters). The attenuation results from each of the many locations are used to calculate a back-projection from which the cross-sectional image is provided. With more sophisticated software it is possible to use adjacent cross-sectional "slices" to reconstruct volumes (or sagittal or coronal sections). The quantitative data reflect the attenuation coefficients of all substances in the beam. In compact bone the bony matrix itself can be isolated, but in trabecular bone one obtains a measurement of not only bone but marrow. Bone contributes about 20 to 30 percent to the total CT number obtained, so variations in marrow composition can influence the CT values.

The usual CT measurements are done at x-ray energies of 90 to 120 kVp, which correspond to effective energies of 55 to 70 keV. These energies are most suitable for measurement of thicker body areas and heavier bones (femur, spine, humerus). The usual radiation dose is about 2 rem, but quantitative data can be obtained at a dose 10 times lower, though images are poorer.

Accurate CT measurements have been obtained on the compact bone of the tibia and femoral shaft; the radius shaft is too small to measure accurately. In contrast several studies have shown that determinations on trabecular bone samples (from the spine and elsewhere) *in vitro* involved large accuracy errors (> 30 percent). This accuracy error could reflect the influence of variations in marrow fat content with single-energy techniques at high kVp. The normal variability of marrow fat ($\pm$ 20 percent) leads to uncertainties of 3 to 10 percent (dependent on beam energy and bone concentration) in the CT bone measurement (Fig. 5-15). The high intrinsic accuracy of CT is also degraded by variations in the composition of bone substance. Osteomalacic bone, for example, gives higher CT values than expected because attenuation by the collagen matrix gives the appearance of bone (Fig. 5-16). This uncertainty affects not only diagnosis but monitoring of bone changes. By careful selection of images, precision of 3 percent can be obtained for both spinal and radius CT measurements, but the uncertainties in marrow composition can double the variance. The problem can be minimized by using lower energy radiation on thinner body sections or dual-energy CT.

Lower energy measurements on the distal radius have been done using specially constructed ^{125}I-CT scanners. The long-term precision of bone mineral measurement is about 0.6 percent ^{125}I-CT. In normal

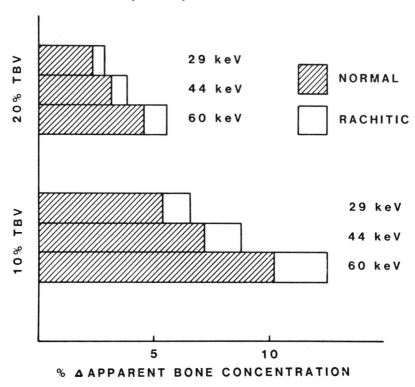

Fig. 5-15. The apparent bone concentration given by CT measurement is affected by the fat content of marrow. The effects of a 20 percent shift of marrow fat at normal and low trabecular bone volumes (TBV) are shown for both normal and rachitic type bone substance. Values are given for the affective photon energies used in ^{125}I-Ct scans of the distal radius (29 keV), x-ray scans of the distal radius (44 keV), and x-ray scans of the spine (60 keV) (adapted from Mazess RB: Errors in measuring trabecular bone by computed tomography due to marrow and bone composition. Calcif Tissue Int (in press), 1982).

subjects, at least, there was a good correlation (r ~ 0.9) with vertebral bone density (as assessed from macerated bone specimens). Consequently, there was fairly good diagnostic sensitivity in discrimination of osteoporosis; the percentage of osteoporotics fell below the 95 percent confidence limit for age-matched controls. The low dose, high precision, and good accuracy of these measurements makes them very useful. It already has been demonstrated that ^{125}I-CT mea-

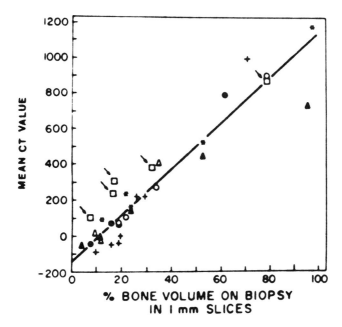

Fig. 5-16. A comparison of the x-ray CT value on the trabecular bone of the distal radius with the precent bone volume on iliac crest biopsy. There is a good correlation due to the apparent inclusion of compact bone (percent bone volume > 40 percent), but the variation about the regression line is high ($\pm$ 5 percent TBV). In subjects with large amounts of osteoid (arrows pointing to squares), the CT values are elevated (from Jensen PS, Orphanoudakis SC, Rauschkolb EN, Baron R, Lang R, Rasmussen H: Assessment of bone mass in the radius by computed tomography. Am J Radiol 134:285–292, 1980).

surements on the distal radius can be used to follow immobilization, fracture healing, and various endocrine disorders. The radius changes in immobilization are smaller and slower than those of the spine in immobilization.

Dual-energy CT has not been used to any great extent, in part, because of the additional dose and time required, as well as because of the inherently poorer (five times worse than single-energy) precision of the method. The precision on spinal samples *in vitro* was 14 percent in one study. Such precision is not adequate for clinical studies.

SCATTERED RADIATION

Several approaches have been introduced over the past decade for measurement of trabecular bone density using Compton scattered radiation. Such techniques have not been very successful, but further research will undoubtedly be done as a byproduct of the growing interest in using scattered radiation for lung tumor imaging. The extent of scattered radiation depends on the electron-density (and hence total density of bone plus marrow) of the scattering medium.

The first efforts by two Canadian groups a decade ago involved a somewhat cumbersome approach in which both scattered and transmitted radiation were measured. Transmitted radiation, at the same energy as that of the scattered radiation, had to be measured in the scattering path in order to make a correction for attenuation by surrounding soft-tissue. Recent efforts have simplified this scheme by using high energy scattering sources with calibration for attenuation (instead of direct measurement and correction for attenuation) or measurements at smaller scattering angles (30°) so that the scattering source can be used as the attenuation correction source (Fig. 5-17). These approaches involve severe technical problems such as multiple scattering, uncertainties of the scattering volume, and uncertainties in the attenuation correction. As a consequence the density values that have been obtained in some studies are closer to those of compact bone than to trabecular bone. This is particularly the case for the approach developed in Israel using a ^{137}Cs (662 keV) source on the distal radius. This method has the additional defect of involving a 2 rem dose.

An alternative approach suggested by Finnish investigators involves measurement of both Compton and coherent radiation. This enables density determination with a single source at a single position. The basic technique can be optimized by using a high purity solid-state detector at a small scattering angle with a radionuclide energy of about 100 keV.

There are still substantial problems with these largely experimental approaches. The precision and accuracy of density determinations is about 3 percent, which corresponds to a density of 0.03 g/cm^3. This is large relative to the total range of density (1.05 to 1.20 g/cm^3) in trabecular bone, and is about equal to the difference between osteoporotics and normals. This level of error is achieved with a radiation dose of about 300 to 500 mrem; to decrease the error to the 1 percent necessary for

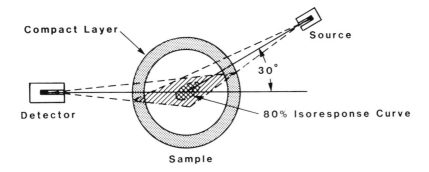

Fig. 5-17. Compton-scattering methods can be done at angles as small as 30° with higher resolution detectors. This enables measurement of coherent scatter as well, or use of a single source for attenuation correction. The active scattering volume may be small, but in some cases the layer of compact bone surrounding trabecular bone (distal radius) will contribute significantly to the scatter peak both directly and through multiple scattering (adapted from Huddleston AL, Bhaduri D, Weaver J: Geometrical considerations for Compton scatter densitometry. Med Phys 6:519–522, 1979).

clinical utility would require development of more efficient (and expensive) detectors as well as increases of dose.

DISCUSSION AND CONCLUSION

It is difficult to assess the best utilization of methods for bone measurement in metabolic bone disease. For nearly all clinical purposes it will be necessary to measure compact bone as well as trabecular bone. Renal bone disease and hyperparathyroidism, for example, are very evident in compact bone. Fortunately, a number of methods are readily available, all of which permit precision and accuracy of 1 to 5 percent on compact bone. This is not the case for trabecular bone. The recent development of noninvasive methods for measurement of trabecular bone does not allow the luxury of use of several methods or the selection of a perferred method in most centers. It is quite important, however, to have some measurement of trabecular bone because of the role of trabecular bone in fracture risk and because of its great responsivity. Where sophisticated technology is inaccessible, there undoubtedly will be great pressures to use simpler radiographic approaches despite their limitations.

Radioscopic observations on trabecular bone have not been very useful by themselves in diagnosis or monitoring of bone disease, though perhaps important as an adjunct to research on bone disease. The chief difficulty is that spine scores, femoral neck or humerus indices, and vertebral biconcavity do not correlate well with the mass or density of trabecular bone. This should not be taken as a cause for dismissing such observations. James Arnold, over a decade ago, pointed out that vertebral biconcavity, though not correlated with density, seemed to reflect the duration of the osteoporotic process. Similarly, the pattern of trabecular orientation in the femoral neck may reflect the duration rather than the magnitude of osteopenia. A high biconcavity index or a low Singh index takes time to develop. This time parameter seems associated with fracture risk in retrospective studies though not in prospective studies. Fracture does not occur immediately on reaching a critical fracture threshold but only after the osteopenic skeleton is exposed to stress over time. Consequently, no single measurement of bone strength, even the most perfect, will discriminate groups of fracture and nonfracture subjects. Obviously time-at-risk needs to be introduced into consideration. For retrospective studies the biconcavity index or Singh index serves that purpose, and when these indices are used together with some bone mass measurement they enable better discrimination of fracture patients from controls. Such indices, however, are not of prognostic value. In contrast, it has been demonstrated conclusively that measurements of bone mass (even in compact bone) are valuable in predicting subsequent fracture; subjects with a low bone-mineral content of the midradius (by ^{125}I absorptiometry) have about three times the risk of fracture compared to controls with normal bone. Consequently there seems little reason to utilize radioscopy of trabecular bone for clinical management.

Several of the current quantitative methods also seem very limited in clinical management for one or several reasons. Compton-scattering methods have relatively high errors as well as a relatively high dose. The approach is perhaps suitable on the os calcis, but not at other sites. Local neutron activation of the spine has an acceptable precision error but the dose is very high. It is doubtful that these two still experimental methods will be developed further. Radiographic photodensitometry has not been useful on trabecular bone because of poor precision and accuracy, but some of the technical limitations may eventually be overcome by videoabsorptiometry. Single-photon absorptiometry on the distal radius appears to be no better than other measures of compact bone in assessing trabecular bone status. CT methods using x-ray sources are useful on compact bone, but the potential errors in accuracy on trabecular bone are limiting and the radiation dose is high. In cases where marrow composition may be assumed to be constant, the method does allow precise monitoring and dose can be reduced for bone measurement. Therefore CT has the potential for clinical application, if only because of the numerous instruments available.

The relatively simple method of ^{125}I-absorptiometry could be used on the trabecular bone of the os calcis with a rectilinear scanning setup. This approach has a fair precision and low dose. The chief difficulty is that the os calcis is poorly correlated to other areas of trabecular bone, thereby virtually negating diagnostic applications. Nevertheless, sensitivity in monitoring changes would probably be adequate.

There seem to be only two methods that meet criteria for clinical utilization—[125]I-CT and [153]Gd-absorptiometry. Both methods have low errors of precision and accuracy. Both have a relatively low radiation dose, which permits frequent remeasurement on patients (and establishment of normative data on controls). Both methods have been shown to be useful for both diagnosis and monitoring of bone changes. For example, with single-photon ([241]Am or ^{125}I) absorptiometry at the midradius, or with radiogrammetry, there is often a substantial overlap of osteoporotics and age-matched controls; the group difference is about 15 percent, or one standard deviation. With measurement of trabecular bone sites, the difference is typically two standard deviations. The ^{125}I-CT method has the advantage of measuring purely trabecular bone with high precision, and therefore may be more sensitive in monitoring changes. The [153]Gd scans, however, permit measurement of integral mass at sites of fracture, and therefore could be more useful in diagnostic applications. At present, however, these methods are in use at only a few centers.

Developments in the field of bone measurement are proceeding rapidly. It is now clear that trabecular bone and compact bone are two somewhat distinctive envelopes with differing response times and sensitivities. As our methods allow closer focusing on specific areas, it will undoubtedly become possible to identify the locus and magnitude of bone changes in all areas of the skeleton. The currently available methods of assessing trabecular bone have contributed to our new understanding of bone physiology. Some can be used together with compact bone methods to improve clinical evaluation dramatically.

BIBLIOGRAPHY

Arnold JS: Amount and quality of trabecular bone in osteoporotic vertebral fractures. Clin Endocrinol Metabolism 2:221–238, 1973

Cohn SH: *In vivo* neutron activation analysis: State of the art and future prospects. Med Phys 8:145–154, 1981

Cohn SH (ed): Noninvasive Measurements of Bone Mass and their Clinical Application. West Palm Beach, FL, CRC Press, 1981

Dequeker JV, Johnston CC Jr: Non-invasive Bone Measurements: Methodological Problems (Proceedings of a Workshop held at the XVI European Symposium on Calcified Tissue Research, Belgium, 1981). Oxford, IRL Press, 1981

Doyle F: Involutional osteoporosis. Clin Endocrinol Metabolism 1:143–167, 1972

Horsman A: Bone mass, in Nordin BEC (ed): Calcium, Phosphorus and Magnesium Metabolism. Edinburgh, Churchill Livingstone, 1976

Mazess RB: Non-invasive measurement of bone, in Barzel US (ed): Osteoporosis II. New York, Grune & Stratton, 1979

Mazess RB (ed): Fourth International Conference on Bone Measurement. U.S. Dept. HEW, NIH Publ. 80–1938, Washington, DC, 1980

Meunier PJ (ed): Bone Histomorphometry: Second International Workshop. Paris, Armour Montagu, 1977

Newton-John HF, Morgan DB: The loss of bone with age, osteoporosis, and fractures. Clin Orthop 71:229–252, 1970

Riggs BL, Wahner HW, Dunn WL, Mazess RB, Offord KP, Melton LJ III: Differential changes in bone mineral density of the appendicular and axial skeleton with aging. J Clin Invest 67:328–335, 1981

Riggs BL, Wahner HW, Seeman E, Offord KP, Dunn WL, Mazess RB, Johnson KA, Melton, III, LJ: Changes in bone mineral density of the proximal femur and spine with aging: Differences between the postmenopausal and senile osteoporosis syndromes. J Clin Invest 70:716, 1982

Schmeling P (ed): Proceedings of the Symposium on Bone Mineral Determinations. Aktiebolaget Atomenergi Publ. AE-489, Volumes 1, 2, and 3, Sweden, Studsvik, Nykoping, 1974

6

Osteoporosis and the Bone Biopsy

Steven L. Teitelbaum

Physicians dealing with postmenopausal patients are frequently confronted with vertebral, wrist and/or hip fractures. The monotony of this syndrome and its association with cessation of ovarian function has led many to consider it a reflection of a single pathogenetic mechanism. There are, however, many senescent changes apart from ovarian failure that may lead to postmenopausal bone loss. These include diminished renal function, changes in vitamin D metabolism, and decreased efficiency of intestinal absorption of calcium. Undoubtedly, other factors predisposing towards postmenopausal bone loss await discovery.

It is therefore apparent that the genesis of postmenopausal "osteoporosis" is complex. Histologic analysis of the senescent female skeleton has underscored the degree of this complexity.

THE BONE BIOPSY

Postmenopausal osteopenia belongs to the family of "metabolic" bone diseases. The commonality of these diseases is their generalized distribution throughout the skeleton. As such, a sample of bone taken from one site reflects changes occurring in the skeleton at large. This realization has led to the use of the random ("blind") biopsy in the histologic evaluation of the osteopenic skeleton.

The iliac crest is the favored site of biopsy of patients with generalized disorders of bone. There are a number of specifically designed trocars available for this procedure, which entails a minimum of trauma

115

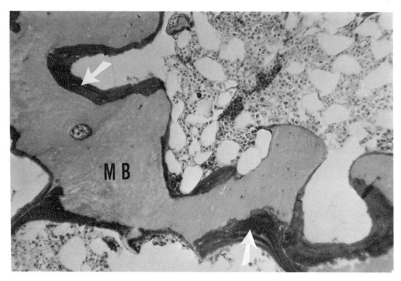

Fig. 6-1. Nondecalcified histologic section of bone containing osteoid (arrows). MB = mineralized bone (100×).

and has high patient acceptability. The biopsy is performed on an out-patient basis using local anesthesia. The surgical approach is generally transiliac, yielding a core of bone that includes both cortices and inter-vening trabeculae. Some surgeons prefer to sample in a vertical direc-tion, originating at the top of the iliac crest.

The major advance in the histologic evaluation of the osteopenic skeleton, however, is the development of techniques to prepare well preserved, nondecalcified histologic sections. In the general histology laboratory, bone is routinely decalcified prior to sectioning. Such an approach makes distinction between mineralized and nonmineralized (osteoid) bone matrix impossible and therefore obviates identification of patients with abnormalities of skeletal calcification. On the other hand, a number of centers now have the capacity to avoid bone decalcification when preparing histologic slides. These methods involve plastic em-bedding and the use of a heavy-duty microtome. The microscopic sec-tions prepared in this manner permit easy identification of both calci-fied bone and osteoid (Fig. 6-1).

The nondecalcified bone biopsy was developed to distinguish os-teoporosis from osteomalacia. Osteoporosis is a histologic entity de-fined as a decreased mass of normally mineralized bone. As such, the quantity of bone matrix per unit marrow space is diminished, but the ratio of osteoid to calcified tissue is normal.

Osteomalacia is also a histologic entity, namely osteoid accumulation due to a decrease in the rate of its mineralization. Osteomalacic bone must therefore contain an increased quantity of uncalcified matrix. Bacause osteoid is radiolucent, the roentgenographic appearance of osteomalacic and osteoporotic skeletons are generally identical. Even the time-honored pseudofracture (Looser zone) is not invariably pathognomonic of osteomalacia. Moreover, many osteomalacic patients exhibit no distinctive biochemical abnormalities. Consequently, the radiologist and internist are usually confronted with decreased bone mass of undetermined etiology and can only make the generic diagnosis of "osteopenia." On the other hand, the presence of excess osteoid is not, even by histologic evaluation, diagnostic of osteomalacia. Insight into this problem requires appreciation of the sequence of bone synthesis.

Bone is synthesized by the deposition of organic matrix (osteoid) and its subsequent mineralization. The duration from deposition of a molecule of osteoid, which is largely collagen, to its subsequent calcification is known as the mineralization lag time, which in man averages 23.5 days. Osteomalacia is characterized by prolongation of the mineralization lag time.

In light of the above, it is obvious that osteoid accumulation may reflect one of two kinetic abnormalities; viz., (1) delayed mineralization of organic matrix (osteomalacia) or (2) enhanced rate of osteoid synthesis. Because the bone biopsy represents an isolated moment in time, it is impossible using standard, tinctorial stains, to distinguish between these two kinetic events. Fortunately, however, the skeleton is the one organ system in man whose rate of formation may be evaluated by a single biopsy. This approach rests on the use of tetracyclines and their ability to chelate newly deposited bone mineral and thereupon, fluoresce.

Bone mineral is deposited at the interface of osteoid and calcified matrix at a site known as the calcification (mineralization) front. The precise form in which the mineral first appears is enigmatic but, within a short period of time, it undergoes transformation into a more "mature" phase, which comprises the majority of the adult skeleton. Following tetracycline administration, the antibiotic binds to newly deposited ("immature") bone mineral and when examined by fluorescent microscopy, the complex appears as a yellow or orange line at the calcification front. Hence, osteoid seams that are actively undergoing min-

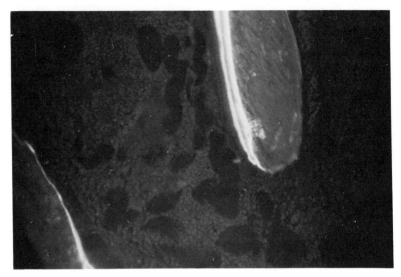

Fig. 6-2.   Parallel bands of fluorescence following administration of two courses of tetracycline 14 days apart (100×).

eralization exhibit a tetracycline label, while the calcification fronts of those seams that are not being mineralized fail to fluoresce. Osteomalacia is characterized by an abundance of such nonflourescent calcification fronts.

As valuable as this determination is, it still represents an isolated moment in time and offers no information regarding the rate of mineralization. Kinetic data may be obtained, however, by using time-spaced histologic markers of mineralization.

Under these circumstances, two courses of tetracycline are given separated by a known period of time. In practice, two, three-day courses of the antibiotic are administered separated by a 14-day interval. Such an approach results in the appearance of two parallel fluorescent bands adjacent to most mineralizing osteoid seams (Fig. 6-2). The deeper label represents the first course of antibiotic and the more superficial one, located at the calcification front, represents the second. The *cellular rate of mineralization*, which is the rate of calcification occurring at the average point on a bone-forming surface, is calculated by determining the mean distance between parallel labels and dividing that distance by the interdose duration. If, for example, the mean distance between labels is 14 micrometers and the interdose duration is 14 days, osteoid is being mineralized at the mean rate of 1 micrometer per day. This calculation enables one to identify the kinetic abnormality leading to various states of excess osteoid (hyperosteoidosis). If the cellular rate of mineralization is diminished, excessively thick osteoid seams must reflect osteomalacia. Alternativley, if this kinetic determinant of calcification is at least normal, organic matrix synthesis is accelerated.

BONE CELL FUNCTION

Bone consists of a small number of cells in a vast organic and inorganic matrix. Despite their relatively small numbers, bone cells dictate the structure of the skeleton by its continual synthesis and degradation. For example, the anatomy of skeletal collagen reflects the rate at which it is synthesized. Normal adult bone collagen is deposited in a lamellar fashion, which when examined by polarizing microscopy, appears as parallel fibers of uniform diameter. When skeletal synthesis is markedly accelerated, such as accompanies fracture repair or various states of hyperparathyroidism, collagen assumes a *woven* arrangement consisting of variously sized, randomly arranged fibers. The structural superiority of lamellar as compared to woven collagen underscores the fact that skeletal stability reflects both qualitative and quantitative factors.

Bone cell functions may be divided into those occurring only prior to cessation of growth and those ongoing throughout life. Growth and modeling are the processes whereby bone increases in size and is sculpted to adult proportions, respectively. Both of these activities cease with epiphyseal closure. Repair and remodeling, in contrast, are always extant. Repair heals fractures and remodeling is intimately related to mineral homeostasis. Postmenopausal osteopenia, like virtually all adult, acquired generalized skeletal diseases, is a disorder of remodeling. Hence, understanding adult osteopenia requires understanding remodeling.

The unique aspect of remodeling, as compared to the other three cellular functions of bone, is its unique anatomic coupling of osteoclasts and osteoblasts. Osteoclasts are the large multinucleated cells that are the principal, if not exclusive resorbers of bone, and osteoblasts are responsible for its synthesis and mineralization. Remodeling involves the activities of both cells.

At any time there are numerous foci of remodeling throughout the skeleton. Such a focus is initiated by the appearance of osteoclasts on a trabecular surface or within the cortex. These cells degrade a packet of bone, forming a Howship's lacuna or resportion bay. Following cessation of osteoclastic activity, osteoblasts appear within the cavity. The quantity of bone deposited by these cells in a Howship's lacuna need not equal that previously resorbed. In fact, the universality of bone loss with age is due to remodeling osteoblasts incompletely refilling resorption bays. Clearly, the coupling of osteoclasts and osteoblasts in remodeling is anatomic and not kinetic. Consequently, a direct relationship exists between the number of osteoclasts and osteoblasts in postmenopausal osteopenia as well as other metabolic diseases of bone. Moreover, any perturbation that alters the number of one cell type will, in a parallel fashion, influence the population of the other. It is this tethering of osteoclasts and osteoblasts that is most responsible for the difficulty of treating postmenopausal osteopenia.

HISTOLOGIC HETEROGENEITY OF POSTMENOPAUSAL OSTEOPENIA

For some years, postmenopausal "osteoporosis" was considered a uniform disease of osteoblast failure reflecting alterations in steroid metabolism attending the aging female. With the advent of the nondecalcified bone biopsy, however, it has become apparent that the histologic appearance and skeletal kinetics of postmenopausal osteopenic females are heterogeneous. Although the skeletal dynamics of postmenopausal osteopenia are spectral, they fall into three general categories. Approximately one-third of patients have low-turnover or inactive osteopenia. Their rate of remodeling is slow, attended by few osteoclasts, osteoblasts, and osteoid seams. Hence, there is a paucity of tetracycline fluorescence.

An approximately equal number have an accelerated rate of bone formation, and we term this disorder "active osteopenia." Their bone biopsies contain an abundance of osteoclasts, osteoblasts, and osteoid. A number of double fluorescent labels are found following administration of time-spaced courses of tetracycline. Most osteopenic patients, previously diagnosed as having osteomalacia in the absence of tetracycline labeling, probably have "active osteopenia." However, there remains a small proportion of osteopenic females who have true osteomalacia. A final third of osteopenic females exhibit skeletal dynamics that fall within the normal range.

There is presently little question that the skeletons of postmenopausal osteopenic females are histologically diverse. The significance of
this diversity is, however, unknown. For example, there is no biochemical test that predicts the histologic appearance of osteopenic bone, and
the changes do not appear related to the duration of disease. Consequently, any interpretation of these histologic changes must be considered tentative.

In any event, it is likely that inactive osteopenia reflects a situation
in which the activities of both osteoblasts and osteoclasts are reduced,
but bone formation is suppressed more than is resorption. Active osteopenia, in contrast, probably represents acceleration of both resorption and formation in which the rate of osteoclastic activity supersedes
that of osteoblasts. Those patients with normal indices of bone remodeling are more difficult to explain. Perhaps they include a group of
women who failed to achieve maximal skeletal mass in early adulthood
and, although their rate of bone loss does not exceed normal, crossed
into the fracture range at an early age.

The variance in histologic appearance of the osteopenic female
skeleton is yet to be shown to dictate therapy. On the other hand, appreciation of these subsets of skeletal kinetics may help select groups of
patients responsive to specific forms of treatment.

BIBLIOGRAPHY

Darby AJ, Meunnier PJ: Mean wall thickness and formation periods of trabecular bone packets in idiopathic osteoporosis. Calcif Tissue Int
33:199–204, 1981
Melsen F, Mosekilde L: Tetracycline double-labeling of iliac trabecular bone in
41 normal adults. Calcif Tissue Res 26:99, 1978
Teitelbaum SL: Metabolic and other nontumorous disorders of bone, in Anderson WAD, Kissane JM (eds): Pathology, 7th ed, St. Louis, C.V. Mos-
by, 1977, pp. 1905–1977
Teitelbaum SL, Bullough PG: The pathophysiology of bone and joint disease,
AM J Pathol 96:279–354, 1979
Whyte MP, Bergfeld MA, Murphy WA, Avioli LV, Teitelbaum SL: Postmenopausal osteoporosis: A heterogeneous disorder as assessed by histo-
morphometric analysis of iliac crest bone from untreated patients. Am J
Med 72:193–202, 1982

7

Prevention of Age-related Osteoporosis in Women

Robert P. Heaney

Prevention is to be preferred over treatment in any circumstances, but is especially important when no generally satisfactory treatment for a disease exists. Such, for example, has been the case with poliomyelitis. Such, too, is the case with osteoporosis today.

Much of the real improvement in health status of the population of developed nations over the past century has come about because of disease prevention. This outstanding record of success carries with it two risks: (1) we may too easily believe that existing knowledge is adequate to prevent other diseases and hence sufficient to extend such success essentially without limit; and (2) we may fail to recognize that the areas in which prevention has been successful have required little cooperation or initiative on the part of those who have benefitted. Even inoculations require initiative only sporadically through an entire life span. The near total control of smallpox, typhoid, malaria, poliomyelitis, endemic goiter, and vitamin deficiency diseases, to mention only a few, is an example both of our success and of the essentially passive status of the beneficiaries. Is it realistic to expect this experience of success to extend into the major chronic diseases?

Knowledge today is certainly adequate to allow substantial control of squamous cell carcinoma of the lung and of emphysema, for example, but we have little or no progress to show in terms of applying this knowledge. Further, we speak glibly of preventing coronary artery disease by lifestyle, diet, and other means, but it is not certain that we know enough to produce the effective control we seek, either in terms of basic causal factors or in terms of eliciting behavioral change in the population at risk.

The status of knowledge relative to prevention of osteoporosis is in many respects similar to that for coronary artery disease. With both disorders a substantial body of population-based evidence exists that identifies likely predisposing and protecting factors. In neither disease have large scale, well controlled experiments clearly established causality or preventive efficacy for the factors concerned. Further, in both disorders application of existing knowledge to achieve anticipated protection requires substantial patient/client cooperation for a major fraction of his or her lifespan.

Even if we were absolutely certain of how to prevent these diseases (and we are not), it seems abundantly clear that we do not know how to elicit the sustained cooperation required, in the number of persons at risk, to achieve anything like the prophylactic success that we take for granted with the major infectious or deficiency diseases. This problem needs to be kept clearly in mind as we attempt a synthesis of current understanding of prevention of osteoporosis.

RELATION OF AGE-RELATED BONE LOSS TO OSTEOPOROSIS

Age-Related Bone Loss: A Condition

Bone mass peaks in both men and women at about age 30, and 5 to 10 years later begins to decline, roughly in parallel with decline in total muscle mass. The fractional rate of total skeletal loss in men is about 0.3 percent per year, and remains essentially constant throughout the remainder of life. In women the rate is initially the same as in men, but at menopause it increases sharply to as high as 2.2 to 3.0 percent per year for the whole skeleton. Certain specific skeletal regions, such as the center of the lumbar vertebral bodies, have been reported to show immediate postmenopausal losses as high as 6 to 8 percent per year. This postmenopausal acceleration of loss in women produces a reduction of total skeletal mass amounting to 20 to 30 percent over a 20-year period. The immediate postmenopausal loss gradually becomes less severe, so that by age 70 the rate of loss in women is roughly the same as in men once again.

The foregoing summary data appear to apply to all races, all occupational classes, all nutritional classes, and to all bony regions and bony types studied to date, at least when large numbers of individuals are taken as a group. Some individuals do appear to move contrary to the general trend for at least short periods of time, but taken as a group, all persons lose bone (and muscle) as they age.

Modern methods of measuring bone mass make it possible for the first time to look at various skeletal regions and even different bony types (i.e., cancellous and compact bone). As a result, it is now recognized that certain individuals may lose compact bone more rapidly than cancellous, and others may lose cancellous bone more rapidly than compact; further, apart from bone type, some may lose more rapidly from certain regions (e.g., the spine) than others. Thus, within the general trend of bone loss from the entire skeleton, we now recognize probably distinct patterns in which certain regions or types of bone are lost more rapidly than others. As is not surprising, these patterns appear to have significance for the type of fracture that may develop.

Osteoporosis: A Diagnosis

As has been pointed out elsewhere in this volume, the term "osteoporosis" is customarily used to refer to the syndrome of fracture on minor trauma in persons (or body regions) with reduced skeletal mass, and not simply to the reduction in skeletal mass itself. This practice is largely due to the fact that patients first come to medical attention because of fracture, and because heretofore it was difficult reliably to detect decreased skeletal mass *per se* in someone without fracture. Thus, for most physicians, fracture itself was and is the principal diagnostic evidence of osteoporosis. Nevertheless, the fact of fracture and the fact of decreased skeletal mass are distinct and ought not to be confused. The relation between the two is still inadequately understood. For this reason it will be instructive to review some of the factors that appear to predispose to fracture.

FACTORS IN OSTEOPOROTIC FRACTURE

There are probably both osseous and extraosseous factors that contribute to fracture in patients diagnosed as having osteoporosis. The osseous factors include decreased skeletal mass, inadequate skeletal repair, altered architectural orientation of skeletal materials, and reduced

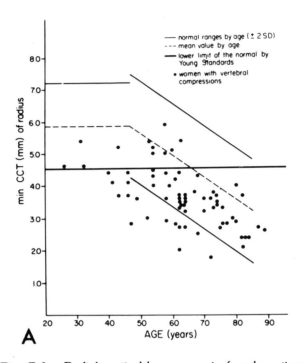

Fig. 7-1. Radial cortical bone mass in female patients
with vertebral fractures (A) and hip fractures (B). Each
point represents a single patient with osteoporotic fracture, with age on the horizontal axis and radial cortical
thickness on the vertical. The 95 percent confidence range
for cortical thickness in a normal female population is indicated for comparison. Note how, irrespective of age,
most of the fracture patients have low bone mass values,
and how, additionally, the older patients tend to have
bone mass values at the lower end of even the age-spe-
cific range. (Reproduced from Meema HE, Meema S: Involutional (physiologic) bone loss in women and the feasibility of preventing structural failure. J Am Geriatrics
Soc 22:443–452, 1974.)

126

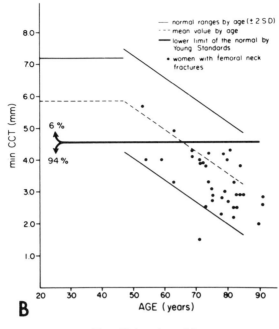

Fig. 7-1. (cont'd)

strength of the skeletal material. The extraosseous factors include principally propensity to fall. The relative contribution of each factor is unknown in general, though decreased mass is probably the single most important factor in most patients.

Decreased Skeletal Mass

The very notion of osteoporosis implies a causal relationship between decreased bone mass and increased fragility. As we have seen, this connection may not be perfect. Nevertheless, it is now clear that decreased mass is important, and probably the most important factor in osteoporotic fracture. All studies of patients with osteoporotic fractures have revealed that, on average, such patients exhibit values for bone mass well below the peak adult normal range, and generally lower than age-matched controls (Fig. 7-1). Thus, as is not surprising, bone mass is a good discriminator between those who are likely to fracture and those who are not. Nevertheless, low bone mass does not guarantee fracture, and some persons with otherwise greatly reduced mass never suffer a fracture. Except for factors such as propensity to fall, cited in the pre-ceding section, no good explanation for their being spared can be ad-duced.

These considerations are important in the context of prevention of os-teoporosis because current preventive measures relate principally to control of age-related bone loss. To the extent that factors other than bone mass are impor-tant in osteoporotic fracture, such preventive measures must inevitably prove to be ineffective.

Inadequate Skeletal Repair

Inadequate skeletal repair refers to failure to repair microfractures and to remodel areas of dead bone. As a result structural defects propa-gate until a major break develops in response to minor trauma. This factor is analogous to metal fatigue or stress cracks, which inevitably develop in most solid materials. Normally bone repairs such micro-scopic defects by local bony resorption and subsequent deposition of fresh bone. If resorption of the damaged area is delayed, however, stress is concentrated at the defect and the crack propagates until the entire skeletal member is compromised. There is evidence that this phenomenon occurs in at least some elderly persons. Vigorous skeletal remodeling protects against this process.

Altered Architectural Orientation

Altered bony architecture tends to be a fracture-inducing factor princi-pally in disorders such as Paget's disease, and it is not known to what extent it may play a role in osteoporotic fracture. One example with probable applicability to osteoporosis can be cited, however. During aging the periosteal diameter of the long bones expands. This inevita-bly makes the long bone shafts stiffer and less resilient; as a result nor-mal bending stresses tend to be transferred to the metaphyseal regions. This has been suggested as a contributor to the risk of hip fracture in the elderly.

Reduced Material Strength

Reduced strength may come from a variety of changes in the min-eral-matrix composite that comprises the bone material—increased brittleness and increased softness. No convincing evidence exists for a role for increased brittleness of the skeletal material in osteoporotic fracture, and this factor is included in this summary only as a theoretical possibility. Softness may be a more significant factor. Subclinical osteomalacia has now been reported on biopsy in many patients with hip fractures. Hence one must consider that areas of unmineralized osteoid may contribute to fracture in at least some patients previously considered to be primarily osteoporotic.

Propensity to Fall

Propensity to fall may well be a more important factor than has been commonly recognized. No studies have been done of postural and gait stability in patients prior to osteoporotic fracture, and for the time being this factor can only be listed as a possibility. Nevertheless, it or one of the preceding factors probably ought to be added to the factor of decreased mass if we are to explain why some people with decreased mass fracture and others do not.

Conclusion

Decreased skeletal mass as a consequence of age-related bone loss in both men and women is probably the single most important factor in osteoporotic fracture. However, other elements such as propensity to fall, inadequate repair of inevitable microfractures, and a degree of superimposed osteomalacia may contribute significantly in at least some patients. Different bone loss patterns probably account for differences in fracture syndromes, but little is known about why some persons lose cancellous bone more rapidly than cortical, and others cortical more rapidly than cancellous.

FACTORS INVOLVED IN AGE-RELATED BONE LOSS

Bone Mass Determinants

Peak adult bone mass in each person is determined by a combination of genetic, mechanical, and nutritional/hormonal forces. Since prevention of osteoporosis consists principally in preserving this peak adult bone mass, it is important to review these factors briefly before proceeding.

Genetic Factors

Genetic differences account not only for overall body size, but for the relative massiveness of the bony elements. Some persons are large-boned, others small-boned. For example, blacks in general have heavier skeletal structures than do Caucasians. Mechanical, nutritional, and hormonal factors can alter the expression of this genetic endowment, but they cannot eliminate its fundamental importance. Thus, as is well recognized, heavy boned persons (particularly American blacks) are relatively immune to osteoporotic fracture, regardless of wide variations in nutritional adequacy and mechanical loading.

Mechanical Forces

Mechanical loading is responsible for variation in mass around the genetically determined level. Increased loading results in increased bone mass and decreased loading, results in decreased mass. As a general rule, within any individual, there tends to be a constant relationship between muscle mass and skeletal mass. Both, of course, reflect and respond to mechanical work, so this relationship is not surprising. It is quite striking, however, to note that despite a 30 to 40 percent decline in bone mass with age in women, total body calcium and total body potassium (reflecting cell mass, largely muscle) maintain an essentially constant ratio (Fig. 7-2). Other examples of this relationship are seen in the hypertrophy of both bone and muscle in the dominant arm of tennis players and in the legs of ballet dancers, and the atrophy of both bone and muscle that occurs on prolonged bed rest, in space flight, and with paralytic syndromes such as poliomyelitis.

It is well established, therefore, that bone mass both increases and decreases in response to altered mechanical loading, and that this responsiveness persists at least into middle age. What is less clear is how sensitively the skeleton responds to differences in activity. It is not known how much mechanical stress is required, or how long it must be sustained, to increase skeletal mass by any given amount above a genetically determined average. Thus, whereas one can safely counsel normal menopausal women to maintain a vigorous lifestyle and to remain physically active, it is not clear how helpful the resultant activity will be.

Nutritional and Hormonal Factors

Although much of the remainder of this chapter is devoted to nutritional and hormonal factors, it must be said at the outset that these forces are probably primarily permissive in most otherwise healthy, aging

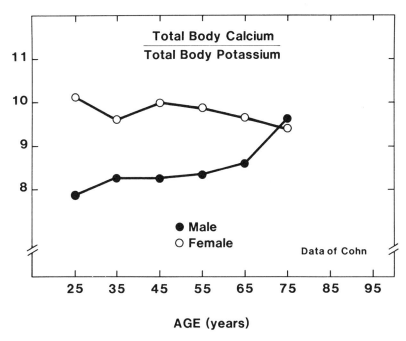

Fig. 7-2. Ratio of total body calcium to total body potassium in men and women. Total body calcium is principally a measure of bone mass, and total body potassium, of cell mass (largely muscle). Note that, despite a loss in women of 30 to 40 percent of total body calcium, the ratio of calcium to potassium remains essentially constant. (Redrawn from data of Cohn, S, by permission).

persons. Admittedly, normal hormonal development and adequate nutrition (both protein and mineral) are necessary for full expression of the genetically determined bone size. It is doubtful, however, that a surplus of nutrients (e.g., calcium) above optimal intake levels during growth will result in significantly heavier bones than are programmed into the genotype. Further, for at least some nutrients (e.g., protein) excesses may be positively harmful.

Thus the mass of the total skeleton or of certain skeletal regions is determined by a hierarchy of factors: first by a genetic program, with variation in mass around that level determined by the amount of mechanical loading, to the extent permitted by the availability of nutrients. This apparently straightforward relationship is complicated by three-way interactions of mechanical loading, internal hormonal environment, and the availability of key nutrients. Three examples, one from each category, will serve to illustrate the complexity of this interaction.

Increased mechanical loading, by uncertain mechanisms, stimulates osteoblasts to deposit more bone during remodeling than had previoulsy been resorbed by osteoclasts. Mineralization of the resultant increase in bone causes a drain of calcium from the ECF and thus evokes increased release of PTH, which in turn leads both to more efficient renal tubular reabsorption of filtered calcium and to more efficient absorption of calcium from what may be contained in the diet. At the same time the elevated PTH levels increase the basal rate of bone remodeling. Thus, a primary, mechanical perturbation evokes hormonal and remodeling changes and altered utilization of dietary components, with the net result being an increase in bone mass.

Another example: decreased calcium intake (or alternatively, ingestion of other nutrients or drugs that interfere with calcium absorption or retention) is offset homeostatically by increased release of PTH, which, as in the previous example, enhances both dietary calcium absorption and renal conservation. Skeletal remodeling rate is enhanced also, but the skeletal balance in this case is negative, unlike when the primary stimulus was increased mechanical loading. In this instance a primary, nutritional perturbation evokes both hormonal and remodeling changes, but with a net decrease in bone mass as the final outcome.

A third example: when estrogens decline in women at menopause, an effective antagonism to the action of PTH on bone is lost, bone resorption accelerates, and it is compensated for by a decline in PTH levels, with a resultant decrease in renal calcium conservation and intestinal absorption efficiency. Once again the net result is a loss of bone, though in this case at a relatively lower level of endogenous PTH than in the situation with frank dietary inadequacy. In this situation the primary perturbation is hormonal, but its effects include changes in dietary utilization and in bone remodeling with, once again, a net decrease in bone mass.

Bone Loss Determinants

The factors that appear to be responsible for age-related bone loss and that predispose to osteoporotic fracture are basically the same as those that determine bone mass, i.e., genetic, mechanical, and nutritional/hormonal factors.

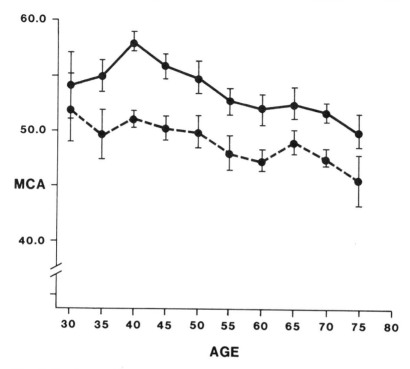

Fig. 7-3.   Loss of bone from the metacarpals in two populations with different peak adult values. Note that both lose at about the same rate, but that at age 80 the population with the higher value at age 30 to 40 still has as much bone as the other population had at its peak. (Redrawn from data of Matkovic V, Kostial K, Simonivoc I, et al: Bone status and fracture rates in two regions of Yugoslavia. Am J Clin Nutr 32:540–549, 1979.)

Genetic Factors

Genetic factors influence fracture risk insofar as large-boned persons are more protected than are small-boned persons. There is no universal, species-wide amount of bone per kilogram of body weight that is in itself "normal" for all human beings, nor even a species-wide amount of bone that is "normal" for any given degree of mechanical loading. Each individual has his or her own genetically determined "normal" amount for body size and for mechanical loading, and it is this "normal" value about which he or she varies. If that amount is large, then age-related bone loss works from a high peak mass, and by age 70 to 80, the individual still has relatively more bone than a person of the same age who started with a smaller skeleton (Fig. 7-3). Thus, although genetic factors do not apparently determine rate of loss with age, they do influence fracture risk because of their determination of peak bone size.

Mechanical Factors

Mechanical factors, on the other hand, are probably the most important determinant of age-related bone loss, although, as we have seen, there are important interactions between mechanical and nutritional/hormonal forces. In general, physical activity declines with age. Even those individuals who continue athletic or other physical activities, tend to be more sedentary part of the time. Thus, integrated 24-hour mechanical loading of the skeleton certainly declines with age, both in the population at large and in virtually all individual members thereof. Since bone mass is a function of mechanical loading, it follows that bone mass must inexorably decline with age. Preventive measures in osteoporosis have to be visualized against that reality.

Nutritional Factors

There is a growing body of evidence that indicates that nutritional factors play important roles in age-related bone loss, particularly in the postmenopausal period in women. Calcium is the most important of these factors. Contrary to older notions, calcium remains an important nutrient throughout adult life. Perimenopausal women who either ingest low calcium intakes or who absorb inefficiently have been shown to be in negative calcium balance, whereas those who ingest more calcium or absorb it more efficiently are in more positive balance. In fact there appears to be a clear correlation in women at time of menopause between level of calcium intake and calcium balance. Further, when a woman goes through menopause her calcium balance performance deteriorates, i.e., for any given level of dietary intake she both absorbs calcium less efficiently and excretes more calcium in the urine. The net result of the loss of estrogen at menopause is thus a negative calcium balance shift, amounting to about 25 mg calcium per day, superimposed on whatever balance (positive or negative) she may already have possessed.

Protein intake is also a factor of importance. Excess dietary protein is, of course, metabolized and either used for energy or stored as fat. In

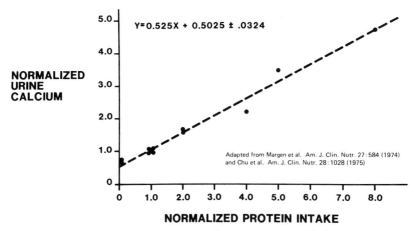

Fig. 7-4. Urine calcium expressed as a function of dietary protein intake. Data for both variables have been normalized subject-by-subject so that baseline values of each variable are assigned a value of 1.0. Baseline protein intake in these studies is 12 to 13 g. Baseline urine calcium is 150 to 250 mg/day. (Adapted from Margen S, Chu J-Y, Kaufman NA, Callaway DH: Studies in calcium metabolism. I. The calciuretic effect of dietary protein. Am J Clin Nutr 27:584–589, 1974, and Chu J-Y, Margen S, Costa FM, Studies in calcium metabolism. II. Effects of low calcium and variable protein intake on human calcium metabolism. Am J Clin Nutr 28:1028–1035, 1975.)

the process of conversion, the sulphur-containing amino acids yield sulfate, which is excreted in the urine. Either the sulfate alone or the associated acid load, or both, are responsible for an increase in urinary clearance of calcium. This results from a combination of an increase in the GFR and a decrease in tubular reabsorption of calcium. (The net result is a kind of biological equivalent of the "acid rain" problem, whereby burning sulfur-containing fossil fuels results in damage to limestone statues.) The effect of increases in pure protein intake on urine calcium is really quite dramatic: a doubling of protein intake results in an approximate 50 percent increase in urine calcium (Fig. 7-4). This full effect is rarely apparent, however, for protein never occurs in isolated form in the normal diet, but in varying combination with phosphorus. Thus, increases in protein intake are normally associated with increases in phosphorus as well, and the effect of the increased phosphorus in this situation is the same as when phosphate is used

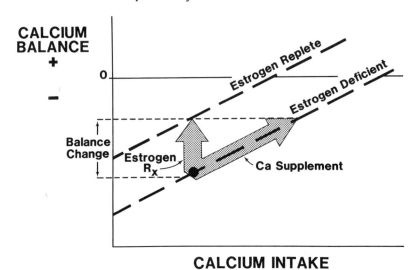

CALCIUM INTAKE

Fig. 7-5. Relationship between calcium intake and calcium balance in 200 normal estrogen-replete and estrogen-deprived women. The lower line represents the least squares fit to the data from estrogen-deprived women, and the upper line, from estrogen replete women. Estrogen improves calcium balance by shifting a woman's balance performance from the lower to the upper line. As can be seen, however, essentially the same balance improvement can be achieved by increasing the calcium intake about 500 mg.

pharmacologically: it reduces urinary excretion of calcium. Hence the phosphorus associated with protein tends, to varying degrees, to offset the enhanced urinary calcium loss associated with the increased protein. Unfortunately, phosphorus also enhances endogenous fecal loss of calcium. The net result of excess protein intake is a distinct tendency toward more negative calcium balance (or equivalently the creation of a higher intake requirement for calcium in order to maintain calcium balance).

As already noted, estrogen loss results in a deterioration of calcium balance, due to both decreased absorption efficiency from the diet and decreased renal conservation of calcium. Available evidence suggests that these effects are due to withdrawal at menopause of a kind of physiological antagonism to PTH action on bone resorption. Estrogen normally serves that function and thereby evokes a higher endogenous lev-

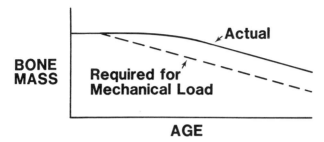

Fig. 7-6. Schematic representation of actual bone mass and that theoretically necessary to resist applied mechanical loading, expressed as a function of age. The difference between the two lines represents the phase lag by which actual bone mass trails theoretically necessary bone mass.

el of PTH in order to maintain the ECF [Ca^{++}]. This higher level of PTH in turn both causes higher circulating levels of $1,25(OH)_2D_3$ (and hence more efficient calcium absorption from the diet) and directly enhances tubular reabsorption of calcium. Thus, when estrogen levels fall precipitately at menopause, bone becomes more responsive to the calcium-mobilizing effect of PTH, PTH levels fall, endogenous synthesis of $1,25(OH)_2D_3$ declines, and renal tubular reabsorption of calcium falls. This explains the shift toward negative calcium balance.

It should be stressed, however, that at least for the several years following menopause the basic fact of a relationship between calcium intake and calcium balance remains intact. Balance performance simply shifts to a different set-point in the absence of estrogen. Thus the negative balance effects of estrogen can be at least partially counteracted by increases in calcium intake. (How both estrogen and calcium operate in this context is shown in Figure 7-5.) The slope of the relationship between intake and balance is relatively flat, however, and thus it takes about a 500 mg increase in calcium intake in the absence of estrogen to produce the same balance change as could be obtained with a small estrogen supplement.

A final word about calcium is in order. The relationship just described is known for certain to obtain only in the immediate postmenopausal years; for how long thereafter remains uncertain. What is known, however, is that by age 65 many persons, both men and women, develop a further impairment of calcium absorption from the diet, and some or all of the ability of the absorptive apparatus to adapt to changes in calcium intake is lost. This appears to be due to a blunting of the response to PTH of the renal 1-α-hydorxylase, responsible for the conversion of 25-(OH)D$_3$ to 1,25(OH)$_2$D$_3$, the form of the vitamin responsible for active calcium absorption from the intestine.

Other lifestyle or diet-related factors probably also play a role in aggravating the tendency to age-related bone loss. Evidence to date is less conclusive, but cigarette smoking and high caffeine intakes appear to predispose to bone loss, altogether apart from their frequent association with low calcium intakes. The mechanism of effect for smoking is unknown, but for caffeine it is known that both urinary and endogenous fecal calcium losses are increased, though the mechanisms of these effects remain obscure.

Alcoholism is also a factor of importance. Alcoholism is now recognized to be a common problem, but too often goes unrecognized in middle-aged women. It contributes to the osteoporosis problem in a number of ways, including generally reduced calcium intake, excess urinary loss of calcium, as well as a number of other possible mechanisms not adequately understood.

If decreasing mechanical loading is the principal determinant of age-related loss, how then do nutritional, hormonal, and other chemical influences interact? The answer is not known for certain, but appears to lie in the phase lag that exists between actual and needed bone mass (Fig. 7-6). When mechanical loading changes, it takes some time for the skeleton to readjust its mass, either up or down. At average remodeling rates this phase lag normally is at least several months in length, and may span more than one to two years. Thus, as we age and place less and less mechanical load on our skeletons, we always have somewhat more bone than we actually need for current average loading. This relative excess may amount to as much as 5 percent of the peak adult skeletal mass, and for an elderly woman, perhaps as much as 10 percent of her reduced mass. This excess provides a kind of fortuitous mechanical reserve interposed between average daily load and the strains produced by occasional falls.

The size of this phase lag (and hence of the structural reserve) is dependent on remodeling rates, however. At low remodeling, the skeletal mass lags further behind actual need, and the phase lag is longer and the structural reserve greater. Conversely, at high remodeling rates the phase lag is reduced, and with it, the mechanical reserve (Fig. 7-7).

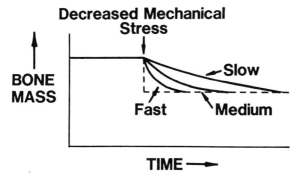

Fig. 7-7. Schematic depiction of the effect of remodeling rate on the time required to reduce the skeletal mass to a level consistent with a reduced mechanical load.

Dietary and hormonal factors play a role in two ways: (1) they help determine peak adult mass, and hence the level from which age-related loss occurs; and (2) they influence remodeling rate and hence the size of the phase lag. Both estrogen and calcium supplements suppress remodeling. Conversely, agencies such as excess protein or caffeine intakes, by increasing calcium loss, lead to an endogenously stimulated increase in remodeling, and hence they shorten the phase lag between actual bone mass and that needed for average load.

IMPORTANCE OF PREVENTION

Aside from the truism that it is better to prevent a disease than to treat it, prevention is especially important in osteoporosis for reasons that can now be succinctly stated. Once the disease is present, mechanical loading of the skeleton is even further decreased because of the disabilty caused by accumulated fracture damage; hence the chances of producing an effective increase in skeletal mass by pharmacologic means are even further reduced. Additionally, once the disease is recognized, supplying factors such as calcium or estrogen, whose absence may have aggravated the tendency to age-related bone loss, become in a sense counterproductive. Because calcium and estrogens reduce remodeling rate, they stabilize bone mass. Hence they impede not only further loss, but also reversal and actual bone gain as well.

IDENTIFICATION OF THOSE AT RISK

Estimates of cumulative life risk of osteoporotic fracture vary, largely because really good epidemiologic data are not available; but it seems safe, from available evidence, to estimate that a white female in North America who reaches age 60 has between 25 and 50 percent risk of sustaining one or more osteoporotic fractures before she dies. Whereas this is certainly a major fraction of the white female population, it is not 100 percent by any means, and it would seem important to try to identify those most at risk so as to single them out for preventive measure, as may be available.

Unfortunately, the studies necessary to identify risk factors have not been done, and the best one can do is to fall back on uncontrolled, largely anecdotal information. Factors that appear to increase risk of fracture, or alternatively, that mark the women at increased risk, include the following:

Slight or slender build (see Fig. 7-8)
Fair skin
Family history of osteoporosis or osteoporotic fracture
Small muscle mass
Sedentary lifestyle
Small peak adult bone mass (ca. age 35)
Low calcium intake
Early menopause or oophorectomy
Cigarette smoking
Excessive consumption of protein, alcohol, fiber, and caffeine
One or more prior osteoporotic fractures

Factors that aggravate age-related bone loss or superimpose another bone losing mechanism on age-related loss include the following:

Thyrotoxicosis or excessive thyroid therapy in the treatment of hypothyroidism
Glucocorticoid therapy
Malabsorption syndromes
Excessive use of aluminum-containing antacids
Miscellaneous disease states, from renal failure to disseminated collagen diseases.

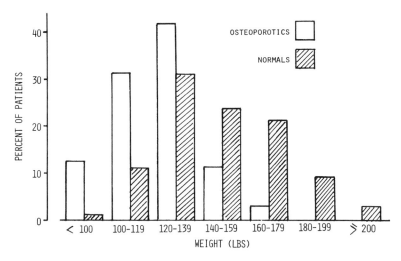

Fig. 7-8. Body weight distribution as a function of age in women with and without osteoporosis. Note the concentration of osteoporosis in women at the lower end of the weight distribution (Redrawn from Saville, in Barzel US (ed): Osteoporosis. New York, Grune & Stratton, 1970, pp. 38–46.)

Although in North America the principal ethnic group affected is Caucasian, it must be said that, world-wide, brown and yellow-skinned persons are also notably at risk. American blacks of African origin, on the other hand, are relatively immune, and among Caucasians, those of Northern European extraction seem to be more at risk than those from around the Mediterranean basin. So far as is now known, these ethnic differences in susceptibility are explained pricipally by differences in peak adult bone mass.

As has been pointed out elsewhere in this volume, osteoporosis is an end-state of many different possible processes; hence there is not likely to be found a single set of predictive factors. Certainly osteoporosis is observed in women who do not fit the foregoing profile. All any set of risk factors can do is place people into two groups: those who possess one or more of the risk factors are more likely to develop osteoporosis than the general population; and those who possess none of the risk factors are less likely to develop osteoporosis than the general population.

PRACTICAL CONCLUSIONS

As has been stressed repeatedly, the problem of preventing osteoporosis is far from solved, and hence any conclusions presented at this stage of our knowledge must be distinctly tentative. It is with this caution in mind that the following suggestions are offered.

For the Young Adult Woman

Preventive care in the young adult woman should be directed at two ends: (1) achieving full genetic potential for adult bone mass and (2) developing dietary and lifestyle habits that will serve the woman in good stead years later. The prescription is simple: maintain a high calcium intake, exercise regularly and vigorously, and avoid excesses of protein, alcohol, smoking, and caffeine. We have already touched on the contrasting difficulty in obtaining compliance with such a prescription.

The need for calcium in the years from cessation of growth to age 35 has, for some inexplicable reason, been inadequately recognized by most authorities, even though the data supporting this need have been available for many years. The rapid growth of adolescence produces what is at first a relatively fragile skeleton, simply because the periosteal envelope of the skeleton has expanded at a faster rate than bony mass could be provided to fill in the skeletal structure. Much reorganization of skeletal structure then occurs for at least another ten years after cessation of growth, and if the adult skeleton is to achieve its full genetic potential, the individual must ingest adequate calcium and must continue to load the skeleton mechanically during these years. Failing these inputs, the woman is left with a small peak mass at age 35 and begins the age-related downward decline from a level of skeletal mass that may be quite inadequate, but that in any case is less than could have been achieved.

What constitutes "adequate" calcium is not known for certain. The current RDA is 800 mg per day, but this figure represents more a political compromise between those who argued for more and those who argued for less than it does a scientific judgment. Evidence derived from slightly older, but still premenopausal women, suggests that the required intake is at least 1000 mg per day. In any event, the median intake that U.S. government surveys show perimenopausal white females to be ingesting, namely 514 mg per day, is clearly insufficient by either standard. Further, what constitutes vigorous physical exercise, for purposes of adequate mechanical loading of the skeleton, is also not known. Nevertheless, a sedentary lifestyle clearly constitutes a suboptimal mechanical stimulus.

For the Perimenopausal Woman

The perimenopausal woman who has a relatively small bone mass is clearly at a disadvantage. There is little or no evidence to suggest that any known regimen will give her substantially more bone mass than she possesses when treatment is started. Hence efforts are necessarily directed at preventing loss to the extent possible. In the premenopausal years this is best accomplished by ensuring a high calcium intake, on the order of 1.0 g per day or more. In the postmenopausal years, calcium intake should be increased to at least 1.5 g per day if no estrogens are used. Alternatively, protection can be more easily accomplished by estrogen, in a dose of about 0.625 mg conjugated equine estrogens, given cyclically. Current evidence suggests that risk of endometrial carcinoma is greatly diminished, if not abolished altogether, if estrogen is accompanied by a suitable progestogen.

Mechanical loading of the skeleton needs to be maintained at as high a level as possible. As pointed out earlier, we have, in the last analysis, only as much bone as we need for resisting applied mechanical loads. Whereas estrogen and calcium can help assure that we achieve this level of bone mass, and slow its loss somewhat from that level, in the last analysis neither agent can cause a skeleton to be heavier or sturdier than required by the uses to which its owner puts it.

Finally, both in the premenopausal and postmenopausal years, it is worthwhile also to control intake of drugs and nutrients that interfere with effective utilization of calcium—either that or plan to compensate for such agencies by significant daily supplements of calcium. Such agencies include, as we have seen above, high protein intakes, smoking, high caffeine intakes, excessive alcohol consumption, and aluminum-containing antacids. Strict vegetarian diets and low sodium diets create an analogous problem for the postmenopausal woman, inasmuch as they are almost always low in total calcium intake; hence they effectively mandate some sort of calcium supplementation to insure an intake in the 1.0 to 1.5 g per day range or higher.

BIBLIOGRAPHY

Avioli LV: Osteoporosis: Pathogenesis and therapy, in Avioli LV, Krane SM (eds): Metabolic Bone Disease, Vol I. New York, Academic Press, 1977

Daniell HW: Osteoporosis of the slender smoker. Arch Intern Med 136:298–304, 1976

DeLuca HF, Frost HM, Jee WSS, Johnston CC, Jr, Parfitt AM, (eds): Osteoporosis. Recent Advances in Pathogenesis and Treatment. Baltimore, University Park Press, 1981

Frost HM, (ed): Symposium on the Osteoporosis. Orthop Clin North Am, Vol. 12, No. 3, 1981

Gordon GS, Vaughn C: Clinical Management of the Osteoporoses. Acton, MA, Publishing Sciences Group, 1976

Nordin BEC, Calcium, Phosphate, and Magnesium Metabolism. Clinical Physiology and Diagnostic Procedures. Edinburg, Churchill Livingstone, 1976

Upjohn GV, The perimenopause: Physiologic correlates and clinical management. J Reprod Med 27 1–28, 1982

8

The Management of the Geriatric Osteoporotic Woman

Louis V. Avioli

The pathologic demineralization of the elderly female skeleton most probably results from a combination of a bone mineral content early in life that was lower than that of males and a variety of genetic, dietary, socioeconomic, and hormonal factors, many of which were detailed in Chapter 7. A number of conditioning factors such as smoking, excessive alcohol ingestion, peculiar dietary factors, and immobilization can be avoided. In addition, effective preventive therapy is available with calcium supplementation in the ovulating and perimenopausal female, and calcium and/or estrogens for the female in the early postmenopausal years. What therapeutic modalities are currently acceptable for the geriatric female during those later postmenopausal years? One should recognize that the magnitude of the age-related bone loss is such that after age 80 virtually all women have bone masses that are smaller than those of normal women before age 45. It is also obvious that women age 65 or older have relative degrees of skeletal structural failure, and that a critical range of bone mass can be defined as essential to prevent the "crushed vertebrae syndrome," femoral, neck, and forearm fractures. The prevention of further bone loss in these later years should also decrease the incidence of fractures in geriatric female patients and contribute to a more vital and enjoyable lifestyle. The potential magnitude of this problem was presented in detail in Chapter 3. Today postmenopausal osteoporosis is a major contributing factor to fractures of the spine, radius, and other bones, causing additional pain and disability in the elderly female. Complications of the 180,000 to 200,000 hip fractures that occur annually in women over the age of 65 in the United States have produced a 15 to 30 percent mortality rate and escalating annual costs greater than one billion dollars! It should also be stressed that during the last 100 years, the industrialized and more developed countries have experienced a decided shift in the number and fraction of older persons in their respective populations of elderly people. In 1950 there were approximately 200 million people age 60 and older in the world. By 1975 that figure had increased to 350 million. United Nations projections reveal that this segment of the population will increase to 590 million in 2000 and over 1.1 billion by 2025. From 1900 to 1975, the population of people age 65 and older increased sevenfold in the United States, while the total population increased by a factor of 2.5. This same segment of our population, as calculated from current life expectancy tables, is projected to comprise from 19 to 20 percent of the total population by 2000. In 1981, life expectancy at birth in the United States increased to 77.2 years for females and 69.5 years for males. Finally, in its 1981 annual report of the nation's health, the United States government announced that nearly 75 percent of Americans who reach the age of 65 can now expect to live beyond the 75th year, up from 60 percent in 1940. Since elderly women still experience lower mortality rates than men, the majority of these geriatric populations will consist of fracture-prone osteoporotic women. What can the physician offer these patients with the involutional bone loss, and what is the feasibility of preventing further structure failure and the fracture syndromes in geriatric female populations?

CALCIUM

A number of cross-sectional studies have shown that calcium intake during early and middle adulthood is a critical factor in the susceptibility to osteoporotic-related fractures in the elderly. Diets with low calcium content (i.e., 400 to 500 mg per day) have been associated with decreased cortical bone thickness beginning as early as age 30 (Fig. 8-1) and a marked increase in fracture rates in the population age 60 and older when compared to daily diets containing 800 to 1000 mg of calcium (Fig. 8-2). The salutary effects of supplemental calcium intakes in doses of 750 to 2500 mg of elemental calcium per day in the population age 65 and older has, in fact, been established with increased calcium

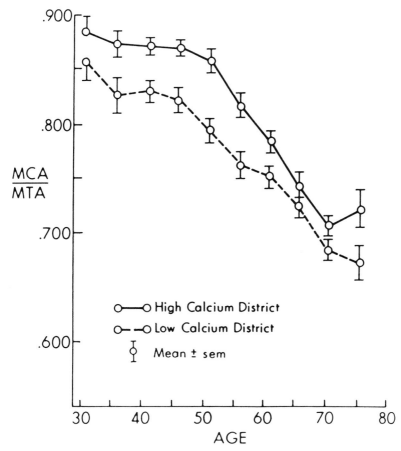

Fig. 8-1. Metacarpal cortical/total area (MCA/MTA) ratio of Yugoslavian women living in high versus low calcium districts. (From Matkovic V, Kostial K, Simonovic I, Buzina R, Brodarec A, Nordin BEC: Bone status and fracture rates in two regions of Yugoslavia. Am J Clin Nutr 32:540–549, 1979. © American Society for Clinical Nutrition.)

absorption, progressively positive calcium balances, increments in bone mass, and decreases in fracture rates well documented. In prescribing oral calcium supplements for the geriatric patient in doses of 1.0 and 1.5 grams of elemental calcium per day, the physician should recognize that various commercially available forms of calcium supplements differ with respect to the content of elemental calcium. Although tablets

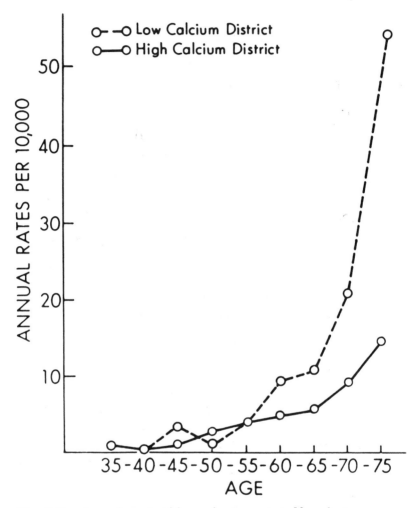

Fig. 8-2. Annual proximal femur fracture rate in Yugoslavian women living in high versus low calcium districts. (From Matkovic V, Kastial K, Simonovic I, Buzina R, Brodarec A, Nordin BEC: Bone status and fracture rates in two regions of Yugoslavia. Am J Clin Nutr 32:540–549, 1979. © American Society for Clinical Nutrition.)

of calcium gluconate (9 percent calcium), calcium lactate (13 percent calcium) and calcium carbonate (40 percent calcium) are all appropriate supplemental agents, calcium carbonate should be considered the more convenient preparation, since the required amount of calcium can usually be supplied with only two or three tablets per day, and patient compliance is more readily attained. Calcium chloride should not be prescribed, since it often causes gastrointestinal irritation. When prescribing calcium supplements, one should also consider the fact that high protein diets and the addition of vitamin D (or excessive sunlight exposure) may result in graded increments in urinary calcium. Thus, prophylactic vitamin-D therapy should be reserved for those patients with osteomalacia. Obviously, nutritional adequacy must also be maintained. This can be achieved with diets or supplements that contain at least 400 to 500 IU of vitamin D. It is also apparant that some elderly females present with blood values of $1.25(OH)_2D_3$, which are marginally low. Although this finding has been attributed to an aquired defect in the biological activation of vitamin D_3, this hypothesis has yet to be confirmed. Recent suveys of geriatricians, orthopedic surgeons, gynecologists, and rheumatologists who treat postmenopausal osteoporosis reveal that vitamin D is often added to the therapeutic regimen. This suggests that a large percentage of physicians believe that the geriatric osteoporotic disorder is frequently accompanied by an ill-defined element of vitamin D-resistance and/or deficiency. This assumption is incorrect. Careful dietary and medical histories and measurements of blood $25(OH)D_3$ should be obtained on all patients before recommending vitamin-D_3 therapy indiscriminately.

The calciuric effect of high protein diets is due primarily to increased acid production, such as sulfate, which is formed by the oxidation of excess sulfur amino acids. Thus, calciuria is greatest when diets rich in proteins with sulfur containing amino acids are consumed. However, the hypercalciuric effect of these diets can be offset by the hypocalciuric effect of phosphorus, which is another important constituent of diets rich in meat and dairy products. Although there are controversial reports of the hazardous effects of diets rich in phosphorus on bone, no influence of habitual phosphorus intake has been observed on the calcium balance of postmenopausal women. However, since carbonated cola-like drinks contain approximately 20 mg/dl phosphorus with little or no calcium, excessive consumption at the expense of milk and other dairy products in the diets of adolescent women who are losing vertebral bone could further compromise the already precariously low calcium intake. Propensity to fractures in later years may be increased.

HORMONES

The role of either estrogenic or androgenic hormonal therapy for the geriatric postmenopausal osteoporotic patient is still a matter of conjecture. Short-term trials of conjugated estrogens in doses of 1.2 to 2.5 mg per day have resulted in increased calcium-absorption and retention, and an increase in blood level of $1,25(OH)_2D_3$, the active vitamin D_3 metabolite. Studies in postmenopausal women between age 55 and 65 on a combined regimen of conjugated equine estrogen (0.625 mg/day) and methyltestosterone (5 mg, 21 days of each month) decreased age-related bone loss. Results of studies using only daily methandrostenolone doses of 2.5 to 5.0 mg are still controversial. Despite sustained increments in lean body mass, this form of therapy does not appear to produce any sustained (i.e., greater than 6 months to 1 year) effect on bone mass. Androgenic agents are probably of limited value in treating the geriatric female with osteoporosis, since the effects are short-lived and the side effects (including hepatic toxicity with hepatoma and peliosis hepatis) are often undesirable. Since long-term therapy with conjugated estrogens may also increase the incidence of endometrial carcinoma, it would appear wise not to subject the geriatric female arbitrarily to indiscriminate doses of estrogens. One may achieve the same result with calcium supplements of 1.5 to 2.0 grams of elemental calcium per day.

The observation that blood levels of calcitonin (a hormone that suppresses bone resorption) decrease with age in females and other observations of a significant rise in blood calcitonin during estrogen therapy have resulted in considerable interest in this hormone as a therapeutic agent in the osteoporotic patient. Although the results are currently preliminary, it appears that calcitonin either alone or in combination with phosphate or calcium supplements can retard the rate of bone loss in aged postmenopausal women. The minimal side effects (occasional nausea and vomiting) as well as the observation that the analgesic effects of calcitonin are attended by increments in blood β-endorphin levels render this hormone promising as a therapeutic agent in the elderly osteoporotic female.

SODIUM FLUORIDE

Beneficial effects of sodium fluoride-calcium regimens on the osteoporosis of patients with multiple myeloma were observed as early as 1964. Effects of this form of therapy in elderly osteoporotic patients have been recorded with evidence of increments in vertebral bone mass on sodium fluoride doses of 25 to 60 mg per day and 800 to 3000 mg per day of calcium. The present enthusiasm for fluoride therapy must be tempered by reports of abnormal bone cytology in patients receiving as little as 16 mg per day of sodium fluoride for prolonged intervals, and others demonstrating serious side effects such as anemia, gastrointestinal complaints, arthritis, and increased fracture incidence. Rigorous assessment of the effects of daily sodium fluoride therapy for sustained intervals in a geriatric population is mandatory before an adequate appraisal of the risk/benefit ratio can be made. Presently, two large double-blind, randomized clinical trials supported by the National Institutes of Health are currently launching a five-year prospective study to determine whether or not fluoride administration results in a decreased fracture rate.

MISCELLANEOUS

Mobilization of the osteoporotic patient is an essential ingredient of any therapeutic protocol, since muscle weight and activity are important determinants of bone mass. In fact, moderate physical activity such as leg walk, sideward bends, arm crossing and chair pull in subjects age 69 to 95 can effectively retard the rate of bone loss. Since thiazide diurectics lower urinary calcium, it has been suggested that these agents might be useful in the prevention of bone mineral loss. However, studies in young, healthy, postmenopausal women who were treated with bendroflumethiazide, 5 mg per day, for two years revealed that the effect of thiazides on postmenopausal bone loss is short-lived despite a persistant decrease in urinary calcium excretion.

In conclusion, it appears glaringly obvious that the geriatric female population suffers progressively increasing risk for skeletal fracture. Despite a variety of recommended "therapeutic" regimens, the efficacy of treatment must be weighed against potential side effects and patient compliance. Since the beneficial effects of calcium supplementation in retarding bone loss has been established, and since this form of therapy is relatively innocuous, it appears judicious to insure adequate calcium intake and/or dietary calcium supplementation until more definitive information becomes available regarding fracture incidence and toxicity with other regimens.

BIBLIOGRAPHY

Aloia JF, Kapoor A, Vaswani A, Cohn SH: Changes in body composition following therapy of osteoporosis with methandrostenolone. Metabolism 30:1076–1079, 1981

Aloia J, Zanzi I, Vaswani A, Ellis K, Cohn S: Combination therapy for osteoporosis. Metabolism 26:787–792, 1977

Doyle F, Brown J, Lachance C: Relation between bone mass and muscle weight. Lancet, 1:391–393, 1970

Gallagher JC, Riggs BL, DeLuca HF: Effect of estrogen on calcium absorption and serum vitamin D metabolites in postmenopausal osteoporosis. J Clin Metab Endocrinol 51:1359–1364, 1980

Harrison L, McNeill K, Sturtridge W, Bayley T, Williams M, Tam C, Murray T, Fornasier V: Three-year changes in bone mineral mass of postmenopausal osteoporotic patients based on neutron activation analysis of the central third of the skeleton. J Clin Endocrinol Metab 52:751–758, 1981

Jowsey J, Riggs B, Kelly P, Hoffman D: Effect of combined therapy with sodium fluoride, vitamin D, and calcium in osteoporosis. Am J Med 53:43–49, 1972

Licata AA, Bou E, Bartter R, West F: Acute effects of dietary protein on calcium metabolism in patients with osteoporosis. Gerontology 36:14–19, 1981

Marcus R: The relationship of dietary calcium to the maintenance of skeletal integrity in man—An interface of endocrinology and nutrition. Metabolism 31:93–102, 1982

Matkovic V, Kostial K, Simonovic I, Buzina R, Brodarec A, Nordin BEC: Bone status and fracture rates in two regions of Yugoslavia. Am J Clin Nutr 32:540–549, 1979

Meema HE, Meema S: Involutional (physiologic) bone loss in women and the feasibility of preventing structural failure. J Am Geriatr Soc 22:443–452, 1974

Morimoto S, Onishi T, Okada Y, Tanaka K, Tsuji M, Kumahara Y: Comparison of human calcitonin secretion after a 1-minute calcium infusion in young normal and in elderly subjects. Endocrinol Jp 26:207–211, 1979

Recker RR, Saville PD, Heaney RP: Effect of estrogens and calcium carbonate on bone loss in postmenopausal women. Ann Intern Med 87:649–655, 1977

Riggs L, Hamstra A, DeLuca H: Assessment of 25-hydroxyvitamin D 1αhydroxylase reserve in postmenopausal osteoporosis by administration of parathyroid extract. J Clin Endo Metab 53:833–835, 1981

Riggs B, Hodgson S, Hoffman D, Johnson K, Taves D: Treatment of primary osteoporosis with fluoride and calcium: Clinical tolerance and fracture occurrence. JAMA 243:446–449, 1980

Schuette SA, Zemel MB, Linkswiler HM: Studies on the mechanism of protein-induced hypercalciuria in older men and women. J Nutr 110:305–315, 1980

Sharland D: Osteomalacia in the elderly. J R Coll Physicians Lond 16:50–52, 1982

Smith E, Reddàn W, Smith P: Physical activity and calcium modalities for bone mineral increase in aged women. Medicine and Science in Sports and Exercise 13:60–64, 1981

Sørensen O, Lumholtz B, Lund Bi, Lund Bj, Hjelmstrand I, Mosekilde L, Melsen F, Bishop J, Norman A: Acute effects of parathyroid hormone on vitamin-D metabolism in patients with the bone loss of aging. J C in Endorinol Metab 54:1258–1261, 1982

Stevenson J, Hillyard C, MacIntyre C, Abeyasekera G, Phang KG: Calcitonin and the calcium-regulating hormones in postmenopausal women: Effect of estrogens. Lancet 1:693–695, 1981

Taggart H, Ivey J, Sisom K, Chestnut C, Baylink D, Huber M, Roos B: Deficient calcitonin response to calcium stimulation in postmenopausal osteoporosis? Lancet 1:475–477, 1982

Thalassinos NC, Gutteridge DH, Joplin GF, Fraser TR: Calcium balance in osteoporotic patients on long-term oral calcium therapy with and without sex hormones. Clin Sci 62:221–226, 1982

Transbøl I, Christensen M, Jensen G, Christiansen C, McNair P: Thiazide for the postponement of postmenopausal bone loss. Metabolism 31:383–386, 1982

Wallach S, Cohn S, Atkins H, Ellis K, Kohberger R, Aloia J, Zanzi I: Effect of Salmon calcitonin on skeletal mass in osteoporosis. Curr Ther Res 22:556–572, 1977

Index

Absorptiometry
  direct photon, 99
  single-photon, 99–101
Active osteopenia, 120, see also
  Osteopenia
Adult bone mass, osteoporosis
  prevention and, 129–130,
  see also Bone mass
Africa, age-related fracture
  incidence in, 60
Age, bone strength decline with,
  90
Age changes, skeletal status and,
  89
Age-related bone loss
  factors in, 129–139
  model of, 82
  in osteoporosis, 124–125
  photon absorption technique
    and, 82
Age-related fractures
  among black U.S. population,
    60
  in children, 54
  correlation of, 68–70
  cumulative incidence data for
    Rochester, Minn., 49, 53
  diminished bone density in,
    62–65
  economic burden of, 49
  epidemiology of, 45–71

etiologic factors in, 52
falls and, 71
geographic and racial factors
  in, 57–62
incidence rate for, 50
lifetime risk of, 46
methodology in study of,
  50–53
odds ratio for, 52
prevalence rate for, 51
prophylaxis in, 70–71
proximal femur in, 54
risk factors in, 46, 53–54
trauma in, 65–67
Age-related osteoporosis,
  prevention of in women,
  123–143, see also
  Osteoporosis; Women
Alactasia, in osteoporosis, 39
Alcoholism
  age-related factors and, 64
  calcium balance and, 138
Androgenic hormonal therapy,
  for geriatric osteoporotic
  women, 150
Androstenedione levels, in pre-
  and postmenopausal
  women, 3–4
Appendicular bone mass
  femoral neck fractures and,
    92

155

Appendicular bone mass
    (continued)
  noninvasive quantitating
      methods for, 73–83
  osteoporotic fractures and, 73
  scan of, using photon
      absorptiometry, 78

Berlin, University of, 100
Biconcavity index, 95, 112
Blacks, age-related fracture
    incidence for, 60
Black women, osteoporosis risk
    in, 141
BMC, see Bone mineral content
Bone, structure of, 119, see also
    Trabecular bone
Bone biopsy
  nondecalcified histologic
      section in, 116
  osteoporosis and, 115–121
Bone cell function, 119–120
Bone density, age-related
    fractures and, 62–65
Bone formation, in osteoporosis,
    31–32
Bone loss
  age-related, see Age-related
      bone loss
  alcoholism and, 138
  caffeine and, 138
  determinants of, 132–139
  fractures in, 35
  genetic factors in, 133–134
  mechanical factors in, 134
  mechanical loading and, 138
  model of, 82
  nutritional factors in, 134–139
  smoking and, 138

Bone mass
  in aging skeleton, 74, 137
  changes in, 74
  in geriatric women, 145
  phase lag between actual vs.
      needed, 138
Bone mass assessment
  photon absorptiometry in,
      77–80
  radiogrammetry in, 75–77
Bone mass decrease
  fractures and, 90–94
  in osteoporosis, 127
Bone mass determinants,
    129–132
Bone mass measurements, see also
    Appendicular bone mass
  precision necessary in, 79
  vertebral fracture and, 80–81
Bone mass peak
  genetic and mechanical factors
      in, 130
  nutritional and hormonal
      factors in, 130–132
Bone mineral content
  in dual-photon
      absorptiometry, 101
  roentgen videoabsorptiometry
      for, 98
  in single-photon
      absorptiometry, 99
Bone mineralization
  cellular rate of, 188
  immature, 117
Bone osteoid, nondecalcified
    histologic section
    containing, 116
Bone quantity, factors affecting,
    74, see also Bone mass

Bone remodeling, foci of, 119
Bone resorption, in osteoporosis,
     31–32
Bony architecture, as fracture-
     inducing factor, 128

Caffeine, bone loss due to, 138
Calcaneus, bone mass
     measurements in, 79–80
Calcar femorale, thickness of,
     19–20
Calcium
     bone mass stabilization and,
          139
     malabsorption of, 38–39
     RDA level of, 142
     total body, 86, 131
     trabecular reabsorption of, 135
Calcium-48, in local neuron
     activation, 105
Calcium absorption
     in accelerated osteoporosis, 38
     by trabecular bone, 135
Calcium administration, in age-
     related fracture therapy,
          71
Calcium balance, parathyroid
     hormone and, 136–137
Calcium intake
     "adequate" level of, 142
     calcium balance and, 136
     for geriatric osteoporotic
          women, 146–150
     osteoporotic-related fractures
          and, 146
Calcium supplementation
     in elderly osteoporotic women,
          145
     need for, 142–143

Californium-252, in spinal
     irradiation treatment, 106
Carbonated cola-like drinks,
     excessive consumption of,
          149–150
CA/TA ratio, see Cortical area/
     trabecular area ratio
Chinese women, hip fracture
     incidence in, 61
Colles' fracture
     age and sex factors in, 56–57
     in children, 54
     hip fractures associated with,
          69
     incidence of, 46
     outpatient status for, 51
     seasonal distribution of in
          Rochester, Minn., 67
Compton-scattering methods, in
     trabecular bone
     measurement, 110–112
Computed tomography
     apparent bone concentration
          in, 108
     dual-energy, 109
Cortical area/trabecular area
     ratio, in osteoporosis,
          20–24, 35
Cortical bone mass, correlations
     in measurement of, 79
Cortical bone status, defined, 24
Crushed vertebrae syndrome, 145
CT, see Computed tomography
Cushing's syndrome,
     osteoporosis and, 37

Diabetes
     in accelerated osteoporosis, 39
     hip fracture and, 63–64

Disuse osteoporosis, 41
Dual-energy computed
    tomography, 109
Dual-photon absorptiometry,
    102–104
  bone mineral mass in, 101
  gadolinium-153 as source of,
    103
Dyspareunia, in menopausal
    patient, 8–10

Elderly women, life expectancy
    for, 146, *see also* Geriatric
    osteoporotic women
Estradiol levels, in
    premenopausal women, 3
Estradiol valerate, 8
Estrogen, in menopause
    treatment, 8–9
Estrogren-deprived women,
    calcium balance in, 136
Estrogenic hormonal therapy
  contradictions for, 9
  for geriatric osteoporotic
    patient, 150
Estrone, in premenopausal
    women, 3
Estrone piperizime sulfate, 8
Ethinyl estradiol, 8

Falling propensity, fractures and,
    129
Falls
  in age-related fractures,
    65–66, 71
  environmental hazards in, 66
Femoral neck fractures
  bone mass and, 92
  in osteoporosis, 34
  hospitalization for, 49–50

incidence of, 54
seasonal distribution of, in
    Rochester, Minn., 67
  in Yugoslavian women, 148
Fluoride therapy, for geriatric
    osteoporotic women, 151
Follicle stimulating hormone, in
    premenopausal and
    oophorectomized women,
    5
Fracture epidemiology, study of,
    45
Fracture risk, calculation of,
    53–54
Fractures, *see also* Age-related
    fractures
  altered bony architecture in,
    128
  decreased bone strength and,
    90–94
  in elderly, 32–36
  in female population, 36
  propensity to fall and, 129

Gadolinium-153 scans, in
    trabecular bone
    measurement, 102, 113
Geographic factors, in age-
    related fractures, 57–62
Geriatric female population,
    increased skeletal fracture
    risk for, 151
Geriatric osteoporotic women
  bone mass in, 154
  calcium intake by, 146–150
  hormonal therapy for, 150
  management of, 145–152
  sodium fluoride-calcium
    regimens for, 151
  vitamin D therapy for, 149

Glomerular filtration rate,
    urinary calcium and, 135
Gonadotrophin levels, in
    menopausal patient, 4–5

Hands, osteoporotic effects in,
    20–26
High protein diet, calciuric
    effect of, 135, 149
Hip fractures, *see also* Age-
    related fractures
  Colles' fractures associated
    with, 69
  cortical bone loss in, 80
  diabetes and, 63
  diminished bone density in,
    62–65
  geographic factors in incidence
    of, 60
  in geriatric women, 146
  incidence of, 46, 54
  mortality in, 46
  in Rochester, Minn., 57
  in Yugoslavian women, 146
Hormonal events, menopause
    and, 2–6, *see also* Estrogen
Hot flushes, in menopause, 7, 10
Humerus fractures, age and sex
    factors in, 54–55
Hyperadrenocorticism, 39–41
Hysterosteoidosis, 117–119
Hyperparathyroidism
  compact bone and, 111
  osteoporosis and, 42
Hyperthyroidism, osteoporosis
    and, 37, 41

[125]I-absorptiometry, in trabecular
    bone measurement, 102,
    113

Iliac crest biopsy, 86, 115
Inactive osteopenia, 121, *see also*
    Osteopenia

Jerusalem, age-related fracture
    incidence in, 60–61

Levo Norgestrel regime, for
    perimenopausal women, 8
Life expectancy, for Americans,
    146
Limb fractures, *see also* Age-
    related fractures; Femur
    fractures
  age-adjusted incidence rates
    for, 58–59
  age- and sex-specific incidence
    of, 47, 50
  hospitalization for, 49
Limb measurements, dual-
    photon absorptiometry in,
    102
Liver disease, accelerated
    osteoporosis and, 39
Local neuron activation, 105–
    106
Lumbar spine
  dual-photon absorptiometry
    of, 104
  irradiation of, 106
  microfractures of, 92–94
Luteinizing hormone, in
    premenopausal and
    oophorectomized women,
    5

Mayo Clinic, Rochester, Minn.,
    53
Medullary cavity area,
    calculation of, 76

Men, humerus and pelvic
    fractures in, 54–55
Menopausal patient, 1–11
Menopause
    age at, 1
    defined, 1–2
    estrogen therapy in, 8–9
    hormonal events and, 2–6
    hormonal treatment in, 7–9
    hot flush in, 7, 10
    osteoporosis and, 13–42
    symptomatology of, 6–7
Menopause therapy, for
    perimenopausal women, 8
Metabolic bone disease
    bone measurement in, 111
    postmenopausal osteopenia as,
        115
Metacarpal cortical area,
    calculation of, 76
Metacarpal cortical-area/total-
    area ratio
    as function of age in normal
        males and females, 125
    in postmenopausal women, 27
    for Yugoslavian women, 147
Microfractures, vertebral
    collapse and, 92–94
Mineralization, cellular rate of,
    118

National Institutes of Aging, 71
National Institutes of Health,
    151
New Zealand, hip fracture
    incidence in, 60–61
Nondecalcified histologic
    sections, preparation of,
    116

Norethisterone, in menopausal
    treatment, 8–9

Odds ratio, for age-related
    fractures, 52
Os calcis, osteopenia in, 100
Osteoblast failure, in
    postmenopausal
    osteoporosis, 120
Osteoid, excess, 117–119
Osteomalacia, distinguished from
    osteoporosis, 29–30, 116
Osteopenia
    active, 120
    diagnosis of, 117
    inactive, 121
    in os calcis, 100
Osteoporosis
    accelerated, 38–39
    accelerated trabecular, 25
    age-related, see Age-related
        osteoporosis
    age-related bone loss in,
        124–125
    alactasia in, 39
    alcoholism and, 138
    biochemical diagnosis in,
        27–28
    bone formation and resorption
        in, 31–32
    bone biopsy and, 115–121
    calcar femorale in, 19
    decreased bone mass in, 127
    defined, 13, 27–28, 116, 125
    diagnosis of, 13–25, 73, 125
    distinguished from
        osteomalacia, 29–30, 116
    disuse type, 41
    early, 14–15

ethnic differences in
  susceptibility to, 141
fasting urine calcium and
  hydroxyproline in, 28
femoral neck fractures in, 34
fractures associated with,
  32–36
and fractures in elderly, 32
in geriatric women, 145–152
hands in, 20–26
hyperparathyroidism and, 42
hyperthyroidism and, 37, 41
inadequate skeletal repair in,
  128
increased fragility in, 127
liver disease and, 39
lumbar spine in, 17, 80
myelomatosis mimicking of,
  17
vs. osteomalacia, 29–30, 116
pathogenesis of, 37–39
plasma alkaline phosphatase
  in, 29
postmenopausal, 115, 120–121
prevalence of, 30–31
prevention of, 139
primary, 37
radiolucency of vertebrae in,
  14
risk factors in, 71
secondary, 39–42
sequential observations in,
  26–27
simple, 30
simple primary, 37
Singh index in, 18–19, 21–23,
  33, 96, 112
skeletal mass decrease in,
  127–128

spinal, 17, 80
thoracic breathing spine in,
  14–16
vertebral biconcavity in, 15
vertical trabeculation in, 15
vitamin D metabolites and, 87
wedged vertebra in, 15–16
women at increased risk in,
  140–141
Osteoporotic fracture
  factors in, 125–129
  and radical cortical bone mass,
    in female patients, 126
Osteoporotic women, geriatric,
  see Geriatric osteoporotic
  women

Paget's disease, altered bony
  architecture in, 128
Parathyroid hormone
  bone loss and, 132
  calcium balance and, 136–137
Peak adult bone mass
  dietary and hormonal factors
    in, 129–139
  ethnic differences in, 141
Pelvic fractures
  age and sex factors in, 54–56
  incidence of, 46
Penn State University, 97
Perimenopausal women
  Levo Norgestrel regime for, 8
  menopause therapy for, 8
  osteoporosis, prevention for,143
Phosphorus
  hypocalciuric effect of, 149
  protein intake and, 135
Photodensitometry,
  radiographic, 97–98

Photon absorptiometry
accuracy and availability of,
79–80, 83
in bone mass assessment,
73–83
Postmenopausal osteoporosis, *see*
also Osteoporosis
as disease of osteoblast failure,
120
histological heterogeneity of,
120–121
as metabolic bone disease, 115
Postmenopausal women, *see also*
Women
bone mass loss in, 74, 79
calcium balance in, 136–138,
149
Potassium, total body, 131
Primary osteoporosis, 37
Progesterone therapy, for
perimenopausal women, 8
Protein intake
phosphorus and, 135
urine calcium as function of,
135, 149
PTH, *see* Parathyroid hormone

Racial factors, in age-related
fractures, 57–62
Radiogrammetry
in bone mass assessment,
75–77
in large-scale epidemiologic
and therapeutic studies,
83
Radiographic photodensitometry,
in trabecular bone change
assessment, 97–98
Radioscopy, in trabecular bone
change assessment, 94–97

Radius bone mineral content
vs. lumbar bone mineral
content, 87
and Singh index of femoral
neck, 96
Renal bone disease, compact
bone and, 111
Renal osteodystrophy, vitamin D
treatment for, 87
Rochester, Minn.
age-related fracture incidence
in, 49, 53
diabetes-related hip fractures
in, 63
hip-fracture incidence, 57
Rochester Epidemiology
Program Project, 53
Roentgen videoabsorptiometry,
instrumentation used in, 98

Scattered radiation, in trabecular
bone measurement, 110
Secondary osteoporosis, 39–42
Singapore, proximal femur
fracture incidence in,
60–61
Singh index, 18–19, 21–23, 33,
112
radius bone mineral content
and, 96
Single-photon absorptiometry,
99–101
Skeletal repair, failure in, 128
Smoking, in geriatric
osteoporotic women, 145
Sodium fluoride-calcium
regimens, for geriatric
osteoporotic women, 151
Spinal bone strength, fifth
lumbar vertebra and, 92

Spinal irradiation, californium-
    252 in, 105–106
Spinal osteoporosis, photon
    absorption technique and,
    80
Sulfur amino acids, protein
    intake and, 149
Subperiosteal area, calculation
    of, 76

Tetracycline, fluorescence bands
    following administration
    of, 118
Texas Women's University, 97
Toronto, University of, 105
Total body calcium
    total body potassium and, 131
    trabecular bone volume and,
    86
Trabecular bone
    aging decline of, 88–89
    dual-photon absorptiometry
    of, 102–104
    local neuron activation in
    measurement of, 105–106
    metabolic disease of, 111
    responsivity of, 86–88
    therapeutic modalities and, 87
    weight-bearing function of, 91
Trabecular bone changes,
    radioscopy in
    measurement of, 94–98,
    112
Trabecular bone density,
    compressive strength and,
    91
Trabecular bone measurement,
    94–98
    Compton-scattering methods
    in, 110, 112

computed tomography in,
    106–109
^{125}I and ^{241}AM absorptiometry
    in, 102, 113
scattered radiation in, 110–111
Trabecular bone quantitation
    locational specificity and, 86
    noninvasive methods for,
    85–113
Trabecular bone strength, age-
    related decline of, 90
Trabecular bone volume
    and femoral fractures in
    females, 95
    total body calcium and, 86
    in young and old normal and
    osteoporotic men and
    women, 30
Trabecular osteoporosis,
    diagnosis of, 25
Trauma, in age-related fractures,
    65–67

United States, fracture incidence
    rates for, 60
United States Public Health
    Service, 60
Urine calcium, as function of
    dietary protein intake,
    135

Vertebral fracture, radial bone
    mass measurements for
    women with, 81
Vitamin D, age-related fractures
    and, 61
Vitamin D metabolism,
    steatorrhea and, 39–41
Vitamin D metabolites,
    osteoporosis and, 87

Vitamin D therapy, in geriatric
    osteoporotic women,
    149

Washington, University of, 98
Women, *see also* Female;
    Geriatric osteoporotic
    women
  Colles' fractures in, 56–57
  hip fracture in, 54
  humerus fractures in, 54
  pelvic fractures in, 54–56
  prevention of age-related
    osteoporosis in, 123–143
  proximal femur fractures in,
    54

radical cortical bone mass in,
    126

X-ray videoabsorptiometry, for
    bone mineral content
    measurement, 98

Young adult women,
    osteoporosis prevention
    in, 142–143
Yugoslavia, proximal femur
    fracture incidence in, 61
Yugoslavian women
  annual proximal femur
    fracture rate for, 148
  metacarpal cortical/total area
    ratio for, 148

a
b
3 c
4 d
5 e
6 f
7 g
8 h
9 i
8 0 j